IOLOMI

Practical Dental Local Anaesthesia

Quintessentials of Dental Practice – 6
Oral Surgery and Oral Medicine - 1

Practical Dental Local Anaesthesia

By
John G Meechan

Editor-in-Chief: Nairn H F Wilson
Oral Surgery and Oral Medicine Editor: John G Meechan

Quintessence Publishing Co. Ltd.

London, Berlin, Chicago, Copenhagen, Paris, Milan, Barcelona,
Istanbul, São Paulo, Tokyo, New Dehli, Moscow, Prague, Warsaw

British Library Cataloguing in Publication Data

Meechan, J. G.
Practical dental local anaesthesia. - (The quintessentials of dental practice)
1. Anesthesia in dentistry 2. Local anesthesia
I. Title II. Wilson, Nairn H. F.
617.9′676

ISBN 1-85097-051-3

Copyright © 2002 Quintessence Publishing Co. Ltd., London

ISBN 1-85097-051-3

Foreword

Painless, effective local anaesthesia is a real practice builder. Irrespective of how confident prospective readers may be about their knowledge and techniques in dental local anaesthesia, this volume in the Quintessentials for General Dental Practitioners Series is bound to provide new knowledge and understanding. Questions as to what best to do, where and when, notably in the presence of complicating factors and in the event of failed anaesthesia, are addressed in confidence-giving detail. The text, in the style of the Quintessentials Series, has been prepared primarily for the hard-pressed practitioner and the student seeking the benefit of experience tempered by authoritative insight.

Practical Dental Local Anaesthesia will give practitioners and students alike something to apply for the immediate benefit of their patients. Whether this benefit stems from a nugget of information or a stimulus to adopt a fresh approach to state-of-the-art dental local anaesthesia, Practical Dental Local Anaesthesia will undoubtedly prove to be a valuable addition to every dentist's library.

Nairn Wilson
Editor-in-Chief

Acknowledgements

This book could not have been written without the help of a number of people. Janet Howarth, Jan Ledvinka, Carole Rose and David Rynn all helped with the photography in Newcastle. John Rout of the Birmingham Dental Hospital kindly provided Fig 9-1. Figs 7-1 and 9-4 are reproduced from *Dental Update* by permission of George Warman Publications (UK) Ltd. Fig 9-5 originally appeared in R R Welbury (ed.), *Paediatric Dentistry,* and is reproduced by permission of Oxford University Press.

The time invested in writing this book would not have been possible without the understanding and support of my family. So to Jan, Rob and Si – a big "Thank you".

John G Meechan

Contents

Chapter 1
Basic Pharmacology and Anatomy: A Whistle-stop Tour

Aim

The aim of this chapter is to describe the basic principles of dental local anaesthesia.

Outcome

After reading this chapter you should have a basic understanding of the pharmacology and anatomy of dental local anaesthesia.

Introduction and Terminology

The main purpose of this book is to act as a practical guide to the use of local anaesthesia in dentistry. Before embarking on practical issues it is important to acquire a basic understanding of the pharmacology and anatomy of dental local anaesthesia. Anaesthesia is defined as a loss of sensation in a circumscribed area of the body by a depression of excitation in nerve endings or an inhibition of the conduction process in peripheral nerves. This definition includes all sensation. In dentistry it is pain sensation we want to eliminate. Loss of pain sensation is termed analgesia. The terms local anaesthesia and local analgesia are used almost synonymously in dental practice. As true anaesthesia may be produced on occasion following intra-oral injection, the former term is used in this book.

How is Local Anaesthesia Achieved?

Local anaesthesia may be obtained by a number of mechanisms. Traumatic severance of a nerve will produce it. This may occur after damage to the lingual nerve during third molar surgery. This is not always reversible. In order to be acceptable for clinical use a reversible method is required. Local anaesthetic drugs achieve this goal. Although the mechanism of local anaesthetic action is complex it can be explained in a straightforward way. A nerve transmits information along its length by producing a change in the electrical gradient across the nerve cell membrane (Fig 1-1). At rest the inside of

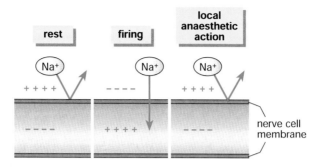

Fig 1-1 The major factor involved in nerve transmission is the differential concentration of sodium ions across the nerve membrane. Local anaesthetics block the entry of sodium into the cell and thus prevent "firing".

the nerve cell is negatively charged compared to the outside. When the nerve is excited to the so-called "firing" level this polarity changes. The reversal in electrical charge is the signal that is transmitted along the nerve. This change in polarity is principally due to the rapid entry of positively charged sodium ions into the cell. At rest the cell is impermeable to sodium ions. Stimulation causes a conformational change that permits the inward passage of these positive ions. Thus, transmission is dependent upon sodium ion entry. This occurs at the sodium channel. Local anaesthetics work by inhibiting the passage of sodium into the nerve cell. In simple terms they act as chemical roadblocks to the transmission of electrical impulses. They achieve this by a combination of two mechanisms. First, there is probably a contribution to the effect by a non-specific expansion of the nerve cell membrane. This causes physical obstruction of the sodium channel. Secondly, and more importantly, local anaesthetics bind reversibly to specific receptors in the sodium channel. The binding site for the local anaesthetic molecule is exposed during a conformational change that occurs to the sodium channel during the refractory period of the firing cycle. During this period further stimulation of the nerve is ineffective in producing a signal. When the local anaesthetic binds to its receptor the sodium channel is maintained in the refractory conformation. A simplified diagrammatic representation of this action is shown in Fig 1-2.

Access to the local anaesthetic binding site is obtained from the inside of the nerve cell. This is important and represents an interesting pharmacological challenge. Why? In order to gain entry into the cell the anaesthetic must be

Fig 1-2 At rest, ion passage through the sodium channel is inhibited by a gate known as the "m" (for "make") gate. This gate is open during "firing". During the refractory period, another gate, the "h" (for "halt") gate, closes blocking further sodium entry. The local anaesthetic molecule binds to a receptor on or close to the "h" gate maintaining the channel in the refractory conformation.

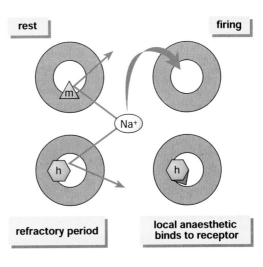

Fig 1-3 Local anaesthetics molecules are present in both charged and uncharged forms in solution. It is the uncharged moiety that enters the nerve cell. This then re-equilibrates to charged and uncharged forms and the charged portion binds to the specific receptor to block sodium entry.

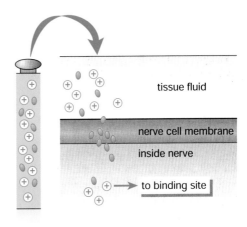

soluble in fat, as the cell membrane contains much lipid. Non-charged molecules are fat-soluble. Therefore, to gain entry into the cell the local anaesthetic must be in a non-charged state. As specific binding to a receptor is important in achieving anaesthesia a material that recognises its receptor is needed. Receptor binding depends upon the molecule being charged. Thus, once in the cell, it is important that the molecule is in a charged form. This ability to exist in both lipid-soluble and charged states is achieved because local anaesthetics are weak bases. When the local anaesthetic is in solution some of the molecules are charged and some are uncharged (Fig 1-3). It is

3

only the uncharged molecules that can penetrate the lipid nerve cell membrane to gain access to the inside of the cell. The uncharged portion enters the nerve cell and then re-equilibrates in this aqueous environment to a mixture of charged and uncharged molecules. Once in the cell it is the charged portion that binds to the specific receptor. If no material enters the cell the local anaesthetic will not function. The more rapidly a local anaesthetic enters the cell the more effective it is and the quicker it will act. Thus materials that have a high proportion of uncharged molecules present in tissue fluid after injection are the most effective. Two factors govern the proportion of charged to uncharged molecules following injection. These are:

- the pH of the region
- the dissociation constant (pKa) of the local anaesthetic molecule.

The relationship of these factors to the proportion of charged and uncharged molecules in solution is explained in the Henderson Hasselbach equation:

$$\text{Log} \ \frac{\text{ionised base (charged moiety)}}{\text{unionised base (lipid soluble fraction)}} = pKa - pH$$

Therefore, the lower the pH the less uncharged local anaesthetic molecules are present in solution. The lower the pKa the more uncharged molecules exist. Local anaesthetics vary in their pKas and thus differ in their onset of action. For example, the older dental local anaesthetic procaine had a pKa of 9.0 compared to the pKa of 7.9 for lidocaine. This is one reason why lidocaine is a much more effective local anaesthetic compared to procaine.

Another reason why local anaesthetics vary in their inherent activity is due to the fact that they differ in their effects on blood vessels. Most of the clinically useful local anaesthetic agents are vasodilators; an exception is cocaine, which has potent vasoconstrictive properties. The degree of vasodilatation varies between agents. Procaine is a potent vasodilator whereas mepivacaine has less vasodilator action. As local anaesthetics have a dilator effect on blood vessels they are often combined with vasoconstrictor drugs such as epinephrine to increase their efficacy. The addition of a vasoconstrictor increases both the depth and the duration of local anaesthesia as well as reducing blood loss during surgical procedures.

Metabolism

Eventually all of an injected dose of a local anaesthetic is absorbed into the blood stream to undergo metabolism prior to excretion in urine. The type of agent involved determines its metabolism. There are two classes of local anaesthetic agent:

- esters
- amides.

Esters are metabolised rapidly in plasma by pseudocholinesterases. An example of an ester is the topical anaesthetic agent benzocaine. The breakdown of amides is more complex and slower than that of the esters. All of the local anaesthetic drugs available in dental cartridges in the UK are amides. Most of these drugs have to be transported to the liver to begin their breakdown. Some metabolism of prilocaine also occurs in the lungs. An exception to the usual process occurs with articaine. This agent undergoes initial biotransformation in plasma by esterases, this means that articaine is metabolised more rapidly than the other amide agents used in dentistry. Very little of an administered local anaesthetic is excreted unchanged in urine.

Practical Points

In order to produce their effect local anaesthetics must be placed close to the nerve they are going to anaesthetise. In dentistry this is usually achieved by topical application or by injection. A sufficient amount must be used, as the effect is dose-dependent. One area where nerve conduction may be blocked is close to the nerve ending. Techniques such as infiltration, intra-osseous, intraligamentary and topical anaesthesia work this way. Alternatively, transmission may be blocked at any part of a nerve trunk proximal to the ending; this is the so-called regional block. In order to be competent in providing dental local anaesthesia, especially by regional block injection, it is essential to have an understanding of the anatomy of the sensory nerves that supply the teeth and associated structures.

The Anatomy of Dental Local Anaesthesia

The anatomy of dental local anaesthesia is not complex. For most purposes only two branches of the trigeminal (the fifth cranial) nerve need be considered. These are:

- the maxillary division
- the mandibular division.

The rider to this is that on occasion some "rogue" supply from other sources, such as the upper cervical nerves, may contribute to pulpal nerve supply. The consequences of this are discussed in Chapter 8.

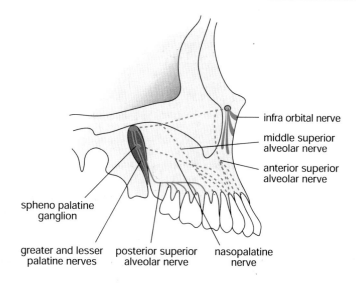

Fig 1-4 The branches of the maxillary division of the trigeminal nerve that are important in dental local anaesthesia.

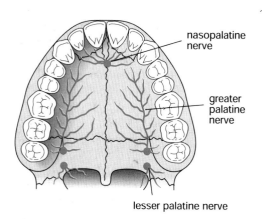

Fig 1-5 The nasopalatine, greater and lesser palatine nerves.

The maxillary division of the trigeminal nerve
Branches of the maxillary division of the trigeminal nerve supply the upper teeth and their supporting structures (Figs 1-4 and 1-5). The nerves of interest are:

- posterior superior alveolar nerve
- middle superior alveolar nerve
- anterior superior alveolar nerve
- greater palatine nerve
- lesser palatine nerve
- nasopalatine (long sphenopalatine) nerve.

The maxillary division of the trigeminal nerve is best considered in two portions. The first is that part between the skull and the maxilla. This section of the nerve emerges from the skull through the foramen rotundum. It then enters the pterygopalatine fossa. A number of branches leave the main trunk in the pterygopalatine fossa; some of these subsequently enter the maxilla independent of the main nerve bundle. The nasopalatine, greater and lesser palatine nerves leave the main trunk to enter the sphenopalatine ganglion. The nasopalatine nerve continues along the nasal septum and exits the maxilla at the incisive papilla. The greater and lesser palatine nerves exit the greater palatine and lesser palatine foramina respectively (Fig 1-5). The former nerve passes anteriorly towards the region supplied by the nasopalatine nerve and the latter passes posteriorly into the soft palate and uvula. The zygomatic and posterior-superior alveolar nerves also leave the main trunk of the maxillary nerve in the pterygopalatine fossa. The posterior-superior alveolar nerve runs inferiorly along the posterior wall of the maxilla to enter that bone about a centimetre above and behind the third molar tooth.

The second part of the maxillary nerve comprises of that section of the main nerve bundle that enters the maxilla. The nerve passes through the inferior orbital fissure to enter the orbit. In the floor of the orbit it enters the infraorbital canal. The middle superior alveolar nerve leaves the main trunk within this canal and travels inferiorly in the lateral wall of the maxillary antrum to the alveolus. At a more anterior part of the infra-orbital canal the main trunk supplies the anterior superior alveolar nerve that descends to the alveolus at the anterior maxilla. The remaining part of the maxillary nerves continues as the infraorbital nerve and exits the maxilla at the infra-orbital foramen. The structures of importance in dental local anaesthesia supplied by the maxillary nerve are given in Table 1-1.

Table 1-1. **Normal nerve supply to maxillary teeth and surrounding structures.**

Structure	Nerve supply
second and third molars and adjacent buccal gingiva, mucosa, periodontium and buccal alveolar bone	posterior superior alveolar nerve
first molar and adjacent buccal gingiva, mucosa, periodontium and buccal alveolar bone	mesiobuccal pulp from middle superior alveolar nerve; distobuccal and palatal pulps from posterior superior alveolar nerve
premolars and adjacent buccal gingiva, mucosa, periodontium and buccal alveolar bone	middle superior alveolar nerve
canines and adjacent buccal gingiva, mucosa, periodontium and buccal alveolar bone	anterior superior alveolar nerve
incisors and adjacent buccal gingiva, mucosa, periodontium and buccal alveolar bone	anterior superior alveolar nerve
palatal mucosa and bone adjacent to molars and premolars	greater palatine nerve
palatal mucosa and bone adjacent to canines	greater palatine and nasopalatine nerves
palatal mucosa and bone adjacent to incisors	nasopalatine nerve
soft palate and uvula	lesser palatine nerve
skin and mucosa of upper lip	infraorbital nerve

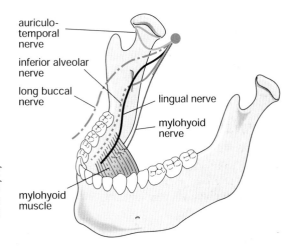

auriculo-
temporal
nerve

inferior alveolar
nerve

long buccal
nerve

lingual nerve

mylohyoid
nerve

mylohyoid
muscle

Fig 1-6 The branches of the mandibular division of the trigeminal nerve that are important in dental local anaesthesia.

The mandibular division of the trigeminal nerve

The branches of the mandibular nerve (Fig 1-6) that are important in relation to dental local anaesthesia are:

- inferior alveolar nerve
- incisive nerve
- mental nerve
- lingual nerve
- mylohyoid nerve
- long buccal nerve
- auriculotemporal nerve.

Like the maxillary nerve the mandibular division of the trigeminal is most easily described in two parts. It leaves the skull at the foramen ovale before separating into anterior and posterior divisions. The anterior division contains mainly motor fibres that supply the muscles of mastication. It also contains an important sensory branch, the long buccal nerve. The long buccal nerve reaches the anterior border of the mandible by passing between the two heads of the lateral pterygoid muscle. It crosses the anterior aspect of the ramus about halfway up that structure. At this point the long buccal nerve splits into branches which pierce buccinator to reach the buccal gingiva. The remaining fibres pass anteriorly to supply the skin of the cheek.

The posterior division of the mandibular nerve runs medial to the lateral pterygoid muscle and splits into a number of branches that are important in dental local anaesthesia. These include the inferior alveolar nerve, the mylohyoid nerve, the lingual nerve and the auriculotemporal nerve.

The inferior alveolar nerve passes between the pterygoid muscles. It travels between the medial aspect of the ramus and the sphenomandibular ligament to enter the mandible at the mandibular foramen. The nerve then runs through the body of the mandible in the mandibular canal dividing at the mental foramen into incisive and mental branches. This nerve supplies the pulps of all the teeth on the ipsilateral side of the jaw. At the midline there is some crossover supply from the contralateral inferior alveolar nerve.

The mylohyoid nerve is chiefly motor to the mylohyoid muscle but does contain some sensory fibres which may innervate the teeth. This nerve leaves the inferior alveolar nerve over a centimetre superior to the mandibular foramen. It passes laterally to the medial pterygoid muscle and inferior to the mylohyoid muscle. Some branches extend to reach the lingual surface of the mandible and may send supply to the pulps of the teeth.

The lingual nerve passes between the medial pterygoid muscle and the medial aspect of the ramus of the mandible anterior to the inferior alveolar nerve. The nerve contacts the lingual surface of the mandible just inferior to the level of the lower third molar apices, often forming a groove at this position. The nerve then travels along the superior surface of the mylohyoid muscle in close association with the duct of the submandibular gland. The lingual nerve supplies the lingual mucosa and gingiva, the floor of the mouth and most of the anterior two thirds of the tongue.

The auriculotemporal nerve arises from two roots. The nerve passes posteriorly between the mandibular condyle and the sphenomandibular ligament to send supply to the temporomandibular joint, parotid gland and part of the ear and temple. Some fibres may enter the bone in the region of the condyle. These may pass inferiorly to reach the teeth by a communication with the mandibular canal or via separate bony canals.

The structures of importance in dental local anaesthesia supplied by the mandibular nerve are given in Table 1-2.

The nerves described above are those that are the most important in relation to dental local anaesthesia. It was mentioned that the upper cervical nerves might also contribute some collateral supply. Cervical nerves C2 and C3, which contribute to the great auricular and transverse cervical nerves, sup-

Table 1-2. **Normal nerve supply to mandibular teeth and surrounding structures.**

Structure	Nerve supply
teeth and alveolus	inferior alveolar nerve
buccal gingiva and mucosa opposite molars	long buccal nerve
buccal gingiva and mucosa opposite premolars	long buccal and mental nerves
buccal gingiva and mucosa opposite canines and incisors	mental nerve
anterior two-thirds of the tongue	lingual nerve
lingual gingiva, mucosa and floor of mouth	lingual nerve
skin and mucosa of lower lip and chin	mental nerve

ply sensation to the skin over the parotid gland, parotid fascia and skin of the neck in the chin region. It is possible that some of these sensory fibres innervate the teeth and associated structures.

Conclusions

- The action of local anaesthetics can be explained using a simple model.
- Knowledge of anatomy is essential for the administration of local anaesthetics.
- Dentists must be familiar with the pathways of the maxillary and mandibular nerves in order to perform regional block anaesthesia.

Further Reading

Seymour RA, Meechan JG, Yates MS. Pharmacology and Dental Therapeutics. Oxford: Oxford University Press, 1999.

Sinnatamby CS (Ed.) Last's Anatomy: Regional and Applied. 10th ed. Edinburgh: Churchill Livingstone, 1999.

Chapter 2
Instrumentation

Aim

The aim of this chapter is to describe the instruments used to administer local anaesthetics in dentistry.

Outcome

After reading this chapter you should have an understanding of the different needles, cartridges and syringes used to deliver local anaesthetics in dentistry.

Introduction and Terminology

Local anaesthetic delivery systems usually consist of these three elements:
• needle
• cartridge
• syringe or pump with cartridge holder.

Those that use a pump also contain additional components such as connecting tubing and communication with a power supply. There are International Standards to which needles, cartridges and conventional syringes are manufactured. At the time of writing an International Standard for syringes designed for intraligamentary injections was being developed. Syringes are designed to administer the local anaesthetic by hand pressure, which may be increased by the use of levers that are found in some specialised syringes. Devices incorporating pumps deliver the solution under computerised control.

Needles

Needles for use with dental syringes comprise of two parts (Figs 2-1a,b). The stainless steel needle itself is coated at the working end with silicon and has a hub that connects to a syringe. The hub may be threaded or unthreaded and is made of plastic or metal. Plastic hubs should be checked for damage

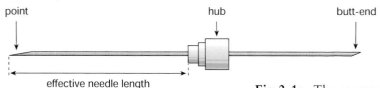

point   hub   butt-end

effective needle length

Fig 2-1a The component parts of a conventional dental needle

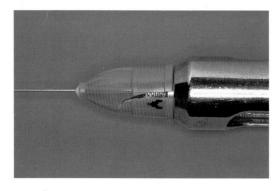

Fig 2-1b Needles used in dental local anaesthesia. The two upper needles are of the conventional type. The two lower needles are of the Luer variety.

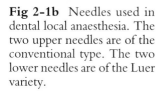

Fig 2-2 This needle has split during attachment to the syringe and should not be used.

after they are attached to the syringe. If there is any sign of damage, such as splitting (Fig 2-2), a new needle should be used as leakage may result. The point of the needle has a chamfered tip.

The direction of this bevel is indicated in some models by a chevron on the hub. Some needles have more than one bevel at the needlepoint and the degree of chamfer varies between designs. The point is classified as either normal, which has an angle of 12°, or short, with an angle of 18°. The end of

Fig 2-3 Conventional dental needles are supplied sterile within plastic sheaths.

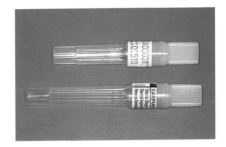

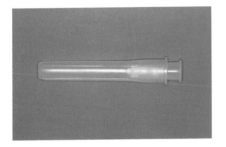

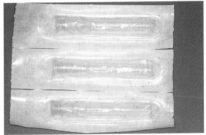

Fig 2-4a Luer type needle with point protected by sheath.

Fig 2-4b Luer type needles are supplied in blister packs.

the needle opposite to the point is known as the butt-end and this has a chamfer of between 15° and 55°. The manufacturers supply dental local anaesthetic needles in plastic sheaths (Fig 2-3). The contents of the sheath are sterile if the seal joining the two parts is intact. If this seal is not intact the needle should be discarded. Information on the sheath indicates the length and gauge of needle as well as the name of the manufacturer and date beyond which sterility is not guaranteed. Some computerised delivery systems utilise standard Luer medical type needles (Figs 2-4a,b). These too are supplied sterilised but the packaging is different. The working end of the needle is enclosed in a plastic guard and this is encased in a paper "blister pack". The contents of the blister pack are sterile.

Dental and Luer lock needles are supplied in a number of lengths and gauges. The gauge is the nominal outside diameter of the needle. In the UK the standard gauges used are 27 and 30. The larger the number the narrower is the needle; 27 gauge needles are 0.4 mm in diameter and 30 gauge have a diameter of 0.3 mm. The effective needle length, which is measured from the end of the hub to the point, varies from 6 mm to 35 mm. The distance from hub to the butt-end ranges from 9 mm to 14 mm.

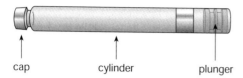

| cap | cylinder | plunger |

Fig 2-5 The component parts of a dental local anaesthetic cartridge.

Needles are for use in one patient only. They may be used for more than one injection in the same patient. However, as sharpness is reduced after each tissue penetration it may be advantageous to change needles after each injection.

Cartridges

Cartridges consist of three components (Fig 2-5):
• a cylinder
• a plunger
• a cap.

The cylinder is made of glass or plastic. This must be clear to allow visualisation of the contents. The following information is supplied on the cylinder:
• contents
• concentrations of anaesthetic and vasoconstrictor
• expiry date
• manufacturer's name
• batch number.

Glass cylinders are suitable for all types of injections used in dentistry. Plastic cylinders should not be used in intraligamentary syringes (see below) as the forces employed can distort the cylinder leading to loss of solution from the plunger end of the cartridge.

Cartridges used in the UK contain various volumes of solution. Volumes of 1.7 mL, 1.8 mL, 2 mL and 2.2 mL may be found. In most other countries the standard is 1.8 mL and eventual globalisation of production may result in this being the universal size. The maximum length of a 1.8 mL cartridge is 64.6 mm; the corresponding value for the 2.2 mL type is 77.5 mm. The maximum external diameter for cartridges including any applied label is 9.0 mm.

The plunger is made of rubber. The absolute constituents of different

plungers vary. Importantly, some contain latex. When dealing with a patient with a severe latex allergy such plungers should be avoided. If in doubt the manufacturer should be consulted. Plungers found in cartridges used in the UK are of two types:
- solid
- hollow.

The hollow plunger is that designed to combine with the special plunger rod found in Astra self-aspirating syringe systems and its function is described below.
The cap at the end of the cartridge opposite to that which holds the plunger is composed of a rubber diaphragm contained in an aluminium metal ring. This diaphragm is penetrated by the needle, allowing the needle lumen access to the anaesthetic solution.

Cartridges should not be used if:
- there is no information about the contents on the cylinder
- the expiry date has passed
- the solution is cloudy
- there is a crack or fracture in the cylinder
- there is a *large* air bubble obvious in the solution
- the plunger is extruded from the end of the cylinder.

If there is no information on the cartridge or some of the information is missing (such as no expiry date) the cartridge must be discarded, as the quality and type of content may be inappropriate. If an adverse reaction occurred there could be medico-legal implications. The same applies to cartridges employed beyond their expiry date.
If the solution is cloudy this might indicate contamination by microorganisms and lead to the transmission of infected material to the patient.

There are a number of reasons for discarding cracked cartridges. Cracks may allow contamination by microorganisms. In addition, cracked cartridges may break during use. This may result in loss of solution into the mouth (which tastes unpleasant and necessitates further needle penetration). Even worse, sharp pieces of broken glass could lacerate the patient's soft tissues.

Air bubbles are invariably present in cartridges. Their presence is not a problem unless they are large. A large air bubble suggests leakage and thus possible contamination. When is a bubble large? If the bubble fills the maximum diameter of the cartridge when the cylinder is held vertically with the

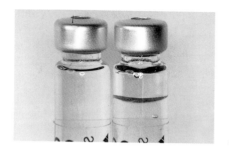

Fig 2-6 The cartridge on the right has an air bubble that fills the whole diameter of the cylinder. This indicates leakage and this cartridge should not be used.

cap uppermost, then it is large and such a cartridge may be contaminated and must not be used (Fig 2-6).

Extrusion of the plunger from the end of the cylinder may occur in association with a large air bubble. This scenario indicates possible contamination and the cartridge should be discarded.

The Syringe

Syringes designed to accept dental local anaesthetic cartridges can be classified as:
- conventional
- intraligamentary
- computerised
- powered injectors.

Conventional dental local anaesthetic cartridge syringes

Syringes used for intraoral injections are produced by a number of manufacturers and a variety of designs are apparent. They are made of metal, plastic or a combination of both types of material. Some are designed for single use and are supplied pre-sterilised by the manufacturer. Those intended for reuse must be capable of sterilisation without loss of function. Reusable syringes must be sterilised between patients. There are a number of universal components in the reusable designs complying with the International Standard (Fig 2-7). These are:
- the barrel
- the viewing port
- the threaded needle-mounting hub
- the plunger rod
- the handle or thumb ring or rest
- the finger grip(s).

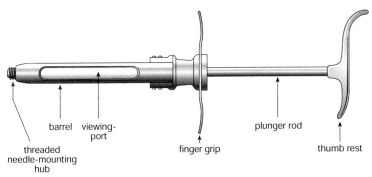

barrel   viewing-
            port

threaded
needle-mounting
hub

finger grip

plunger rod

thumb rest

Fig 2-7 The component parts of a dental local anaesthetic syringe.

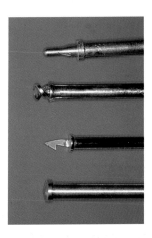

Fig 2-8 Different types of plunger rod ends. From the top these are the Astra self-aspirating design, two examples of positive aspirating rods and a butt-ended rod.

The barrel is the part that accepts the cartridge. This may be loaded from the end (breech-loading) or from the side of the barrel. The barrel has a viewing port to allow visualisation of the contents of the cartridge during use.

The threaded needle-mounting hub is at one end of the barrel. The threaded screw is designed to firmly engage the needle hub. The syringe should be discarded if wear of these threads prevents secure retention of the needle.

The plunger rod has a handle or thumb-ring at one end. It transmits force from the operator's thumb to the cartridge plunger to allow injection. The plunger rod end design varies (Fig 2-8). It may be:
• butt-ended
• have a plunger-engaging device
• be of the Astra self-aspirating design.

19

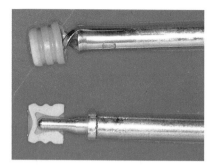

Fig 2- 9 The upper part of the figure shows the interplay between a positive aspirating syringe plunger rod and bung. The lower part of the figure shows the relationship between the Astra self-aspirating plunger and plunger rod. Deflection and then release of the diaphragm at the base of the plunger effects aspiration.

These different designs relate to the mechanism of aspiration. Aspiration is a technique that allows material at the tip of the syringe to be drawn into the cartridge before and during injection. It is an important manœuvre as it aids in determining whether or not the tip of the needle is in a blood vessel at the time of injection. Intravascular injections should be avoided during local anaesthesia for reasons discussed in the Chapter 7. Aspiration can be achieved by two methods in dental local anaesthetic cartridges. These are:
• by withdrawal of the plunger away from the needle
• by deflection of a diaphragm in the cartridge plunger or cap.

Syringes may be classified in relation to aspiration as:
• non-aspirating
• positive aspirating
• passive aspirating.

Non-aspirating syringes should not be used for infiltration or regional block injections, as it is not possible to determine if the tip of the needle is in a vein at the time of injection. Removing the pressure from the plunger rod may allow entry of blood into the cartridge if the tip of the needle is in an artery due to the pressure at this side of the circulation. Intra-arterial penetration is not as common as intravenous entry. Release of pressure from the plunger rod will not effect aspiration in non-aspirating systems when the point of the needle is in a vein. Therefore, non-aspirating syringes cannot be recommended.

Positive aspirating systems rely upon an active movement by the operator. The simplest method is withdrawal of the plunger rod that is connected to the cartridge plunger by an engaging device such as a barb or hook (Fig 2-9). Pulling back the rod withdraws the plunger thus reducing the pressure

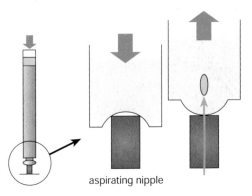

Fig 2-10 The mechanism of action of the aspirating nipple found at the base of some types of syringe. This device deflects the diaphragm at the cap end of the cartridge to effect aspiration.

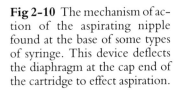

aspirating nipple

in the cartridge and allowing entry of material from the site of injection into the cylinder. Although it is simple, this is a clumsy manœuvre. Movement of the needle tip during this action may mean that the site of aspiration is not the site of eventual injection.

One design of positive aspirating syringe involves depression of the cartridge on to an aspirating nipple (Fig 2-10) at the hub end of the syringe by pressure on a thumb-ring close to the finger rests on the barrel. This ring contacts the cylinder at the plunger end and pushes the entire cartridge down onto the nipple, which indents the rubber diaphragm in the cap. When pressure is released from the thumb-ring the diaphragm returns to its original position with a resultant decrease in the pressure within the cylinder, which "sucks" material from the needle into the cartridge.

Passive aspirating systems involve minimal movement of the operator's thumb and this reduces the chances of the needle tip changing position during the aspiration action. A variety of designs allow this method of aspiration. One method employs the nipple at the hub of the syringe described above. This time the aspiration force is not provided by pushing the cartridge onto the nipple by pressure from a separate thumb-ring but by advancing the cartridge onto the aspirating device by the pressure applied to the plunger via the plunger rod. When this pressure is released the cartridge bounces back on the nipple effecting aspiration.

Another method is that found in the Astra self-aspirating system. This depends upon interplay between the customised plunger and plunger rod in

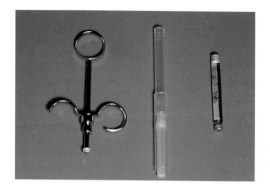

Fig 2-11 Disposable syringes contain plastic components that are for single use. This type incorporates a protective sleeve for the needle.

this design (Fig 2-9). The plunger rod has an extension, which enters the hollow end of the plunger in the specialised cartridges. Light pressure on the plunger rod extends the diaphragm at the end of the hollow plunger into the anaesthetic solution before the main body of the plunger rod engages the periphery of the plunger. When thumb pressure is released the diaphragm returns to its original position and this action draws material at the tip of the needle into the cylinder.

Some syringes incorporate both of the passive aspirating techniques described above - namely, they use both the Astra plunger rod and the nipple at the hub.

Single-use syringes

Disposable syringes for single use are usually made of plastic. Some are part disposable but with some reusable components. The throwaway portion is plastic and the reusable part metal. Some of these designs include devices that are intended to reduce the chances of needle-stick injury during disposal (Fig 2-11). In some of these latter types the needle is an integral part of the system and is pre-attached by the manufacturer. A protective sheath is incorporated into the barrel of the syringe and this is slid over the needle at the end of the injection. This means that the needle does not have to be removed. This has been shown to reduce the number of needle-stick injuries to dental personnel.

Intraligamentary syringes

Syringes designed for intraligamentary or periodontal ligament injections employ conventional dental needles and cartridges. Some will only accept 1.8 mL cartridges. These devices have many of the components that were

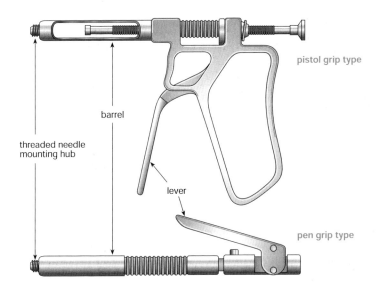

Fig 2-12 Two different designs of intraligamentary syringe are available; these are pistol and pen grips.

detailed above for conventional cartridge syringes. They differ from the conventional type in that the design provides a mechanical advantage. In other words, the force applied by the operator's thumb or finger is increased when it is delivered to the cartridge plunger. This is achieved by a lever. Depending upon the design, this mechanical advantage may be as much as twelvefold. Two designs are recognised (Fig 2-12):

• pen grip type
• pistol grip type.

The pistol grip provides a greater mechanical advantage but has a more aggressive appearance. Not all intraligamentary syringe barrels have a viewing port. When a viewing port is provided it is important to cover the cartridge with a protective sheath as the pressures created during intraligamentary injections can fracture the cartridge. The protective sheath protects the patient and the operator from damage produced by sharp pieces of glass. As mentioned above, plastic cartridges should not be used with these syringes as they can distort under the pressures generated.

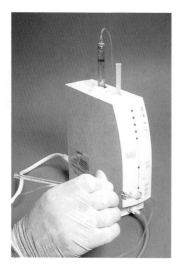 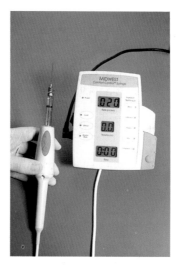

Fig 2-13 The Wand computerised delivery system.

Fig 2-14 The Comfort Control™ syringe system is an example of a computerised delivery design.

Computerised Delivery Systems

During the last decade the design of dental local anaesthetic syringes has been revolutionised with the advent of computerised delivery systems. These devices permit slow delivery of solution. At present there are two designs available. These are the Wand (Fig 2-13) and the Comfort Control™ syringe (Fig 2-14).

The Wand operates by the computer component driving a plunger rod into the local anaesthetic cartridge at slow speed. This allows a very slow rate of deposition of solution into the tissues. A foot pump controls the injection. Gentle pressure on the foot pump expresses solution at the rate determined by the computer; firm pressure increases this speed two-fold. The system accepts 1.8 mL dental local anaesthetic cartridges but requires Luer lock needles. The Wand aspirates by releasing pressure from the foot pump. This pulls the plunger rod away from the cartridge plunger and creates a vacuum above the plunger. This results in the plunger being withdrawn away from the needle effecting aspiration.

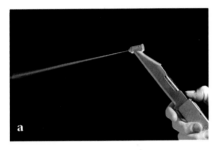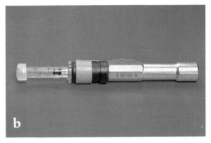

Fig 2-15 Jet injectors force the solution through mucosa under pressure. Some designs incorporate dental local anaesthetic cartridges (Fig 2-15a); in others the solution is drawn up into a vial in the injector (Fig 2-15b).

The Comfort Control™ syringe uses both dental cartridges and dental needles. It has a speed selector with pre-programmed injection rates for infiltration (0.017 mL/sec), regional block (0.02 mL/sec), palatal (0.008mL/sec), intraligamentary (0.007 mL/sec) and intraosseous (0.02 mL/sec) injections. During the first ten seconds of the injection the rate is identical for all techniques. Then the predetermined speed kicks in. As is the case with the Wand, the speed selected can be increased. In this case by pressing a button on the hand-held section of the device. The Comfort Control™ syringe aspirates by using a plunger-engaging device to draw the plunger back along the cylinder to reduce cartridge pressure. Pressing a button on the hand held device produces this reverse movement.

Powered injectors
There are designs of syringe that force local anaesthetic through mucosa without the use of a needle (Figs 2-15a,b). Some, such as jet injectors, use dental local anaesthetic cartridges; others rely on local anaesthetic powder. The power used to force the anaesthetic from the device through mucosa is generated mechanically by springs or by gas pressure. These designs have not received universal acceptance in dentistry but advances in this field, which could lead to the elimination of needles from the local anaesthetic armamentarium, should be welcomed.

Medical Syringes

The syringes discussed above are those that are used routinely. In rare cases where this type of equipment cannot be used - for example, when the desired drug is not available in a dental local anaesthetic cartridge - it is possible to draw up and inject solutions with conventional medical (Luer lock) syringes.

Conclusions

* Dental injection systems comprise of three basic components
  - needles
  - cartridges
  - syringes
* Syringes can be manual or computerised
* Syringes effect aspiration by a variety of methods
* Specialised syringes are available for:
  - intraligamentary injections
  - needle-free administration.

Further Reading

International Standard ISO11499. Dental Cartridges for Local Anaesthetics. London: British Standards Institution.

International Standard ISO7885. Sterile Dental Injection Needles for Single Use. London: British Standards Institution.

International Standard ISO9997. Dental Cartridge Syringes. London: British Standards Institution.

Chapter 3
Local Anaesthetic Drugs

Aim

The aim of this chapter is to describe the drugs that are used during dental local anaesthesia.

Outcome

After reading this chapter you should have an understanding of the drugs used in dental local anaesthesia and be able to determine the most appropriate choice for particular treatments in individual patients.

Introduction and Terminology

Two classes of drugs are encountered during dental local anaesthesia. These are the anaesthetic agents and vasoconstrictors. Various combinations are available in the UK in dental cartridges (Table 3-1).

Local anaesthetic drugs are classified by their chemical structure. Two types are used:
• amides
• esters.

Table 3-1. **Local anaesthetic/vasoconstrictor combinations available in dental local anaesthetic cartridges in the UK.**

	Vasoconstrictor-free	With epinephrine	With felypressin
Local anaesthetic			
Lidocaine	+	+	
Prilocaine	+		+
Mepivacaine	+	+	
Articaine		+	

+ = combination available

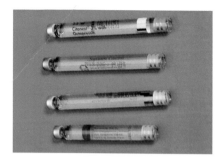

Fig 3-1 Some of the different types of cartridges of dental local anaesthetics available in the UK.

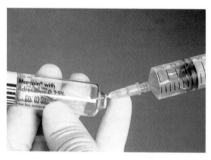

Fig 3-2 Some local anaesthetics are unavailable in cartridges in the UK and therefore must be drawn up from vials.

Similarly, vasoconstrictors are classified into two groups. These are:
- catecholamines
- synthetic polypeptides.

In addition to the anaesthetic agent and the vasoconstrictor, the local anaesthetic solution contains other ingredients. As well as the solvent, which is Ringer's solution, epinephrine- (adrenaline-)containing solutions include a reducing agent to prevent loss of properties of the catecholamine. Previously, local anaesthetics had preservatives such as para-amino-benzoic acid included. These days most solutions are preservative-free.

Amide Local Anaesthetics

The amide local anaesthetics that may be used in dentistry in the UK are:
- lidocaine (lignocaine)
- prilocaine
- mepivacaine
- articaine
- bupivacaine and levobupivacaine
- ropivacaine.

These are the approved non-proprietary names of the agents. Table 3-2 relates proprietary names to the approved version. At the time of writing, only the first four were available in dental local anaesthetic cartridges in the UK (Fig 3-1). Bupivacaine, levobupivacaine and ropivacaine anaesthetic solutions are supplied in standard hospital type vials. Therefore, they must be "drawn up" (Fig 3-2).

Table 3-2. **Proprietary names of local anaesthetics in the UK.**

Proprietary name	Approved name
Chirocaine	Levobupivacaine
Citanest	Prilocaine
Lignospan	Lidocaine
Lignostab	Lidocaine
Marcain	Bupivacaine
Naropin	Ropivacaine
Scandonest	Mepivacaine
Septanest	Articaine
Xylocaine	Lidocaine
Xylotox	Lidocaine

The amide anaesthetics are the group almost exclusively used for injection in modern dentistry. In addition to having physicochemical properties, which confer a better anaesthetic profile than the esters, an important attribute of the amide group is the low potential for producing allergic reactions. Ester local anaesthetics are more likely to induce allergy.

Lidocaine
Lidocaine is the "gold standard" local anaesthetic drug. It has been used in dental anaesthesia for over 50 years (Fig 3-3). When used for injection in dentistry it is provided as a 2% solution (20 mg/mL). Like all the other in-

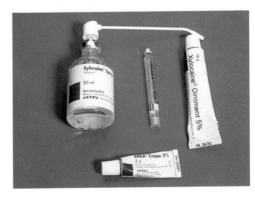

Fig 3-3 Lidocaine is available in a number of formulations for injection and topical use.

jectable agents described it is dissolved in solution as the hydrochloride salt. When used as a topical anaesthetic, a number of formulations and concentrations have been employed - for example, a 5% gel, a 10% spray or up to 20% incorporated into an adhesive patch.

Lidocaine, when used alone, does not provide long-lasting pulpal anaesthesia. When combined with epinephrine, reliable dental anaesthesia is achieved after injection by any of the standard methods described later in this book. The plain solution can provide soft tissue anaesthesia, although the duration is less than that obtained when a vasoconstrictor is included in the formulation. In the UK 2% lidocaine is normally combined with epinephrine in a concentration of 1:80,000 (12.5µg/mL). When used in infiltration and regional block anaesthesia, lidocaine with epinephrine can produce pulpal anaesthesia of about 45 minutes. Soft tissue anaesthesia lasts longer and altered soft tissue sensation may be present for 2 to 3 hours. When used for intraligamentary anaesthesia the mean duration of pulpal anaesthesia for single rooted teeth is about 15 minutes.

Prilocaine

Prilocaine is supplied in two forms in dental cartridges in the UK. First, it is produced as a 3% (30 mg/mL) solution in combination with the synthetic polypeptide vasoconstrictor felypressin (octapressin). Secondly, it is available as a plain 4% (40 mg/mL) solution. The prilocaine/felypressin combination has a similar spectrum of activity to lidocaine with epinephrine when used during infiltration and regional block anaesthesia. It is not as potent during intraligamentary anaesthesia and is less effective in controlling haemorrhage than the catecholamine-containing combination.

Prilocaine produces less vasodilation than lidocaine. Therefore the plain prilocaine presentation is useful if a vasoconstrictor-free drug is required.

Prilocaine is combined with lidocaine in the topical anaesthetic EMLA (Fig 3-4). In this preparation both agents are present in a concentration of 2.5%. This formulation is useful in obtaining skin anaesthesia prior to venous cannulation for sedation or general anaesthesia. At present it is not licensed for intraoral use.

Mepivacaine

Mepivacaine is supplied in two formulations in the UK. First, as a 2% (20 mg/mL) solution with 1:100,000 (10 µg/mL) epinephrine. Secondly, there is a 3% (30 mg/mL) plain solution. Mepivacaine with epinephrine performs

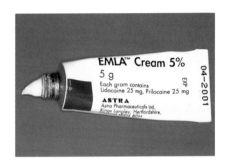

Fig 3-4 EMLA is a mixture of prilocaine and lidocaine and is used for topical anaesthesia of the skin.

similarly to lidocaine with epinephrine. The plain solution is useful if a vasoconstrictor-free anaesthetic is required. Mepivacaine produces less vasodilation than lidocaine.

Articaine

Articaine is available as a 4% (40 mg/mL) solution. It is combined with 1:100,000 (10 μg/mL) and 1:200,000 (5 μg/mL) epinephrine. The performance of articaine with epinephrine is similar to that of lidocaine with epinephrine. This drug is metabolised more quickly than any of the other agents used in dental local anaesthesia, which is an advantage in relation to toxicity if repeat injections are required during a long procedure. Agents such as lidocaine and prilocaine have half-lives of around 90 minutes. The half-life of articaine is about 20 minutes. This is due to the fact that the latter drug is partly metabolised in plasma.

Bupivacaine and levobupivacaine

Bupivacaine is one of the so-called "long-acting" local anaesthetics. Levobupivacaine is the pure l-isomer of the former drug, which is a racemic mixture of the levo and dextro forms. Levobupivacaine is less cardiotoxic than the parent drug. Bupivacaine is available in ampoules in a variety of concentrations ranging form 0.25% (2.5 mg/mL) to 0.75% (7.5 mg/mL) with and without epinephrine at a concentration of 1:200,000 (5 μg/mL). In dentistry the concentrations used are 0.25-0.5%. Similarly, levo-bupivacaine is presented as 0.25-0.75% solutions.

The property that confers long-lasting anaesthesia is that of protein binding. Bupivacaine is highly attached to protein; 96% of the drug is bound compared to 64% for lidocaine. The protein-bound fraction provides a reservoir of activity that can be used to replenish a drug that is being absorbed into the circulation and metabolised. It is important to point out that these drugs will

31

only provide long-lasting anaesthesia when injected as a regional block. When used for infiltration anaesthesia they offer no advantages over lidocaine with epinephrine other than a reduction in epinephrine concentration. Indeed, pulpal anaesthesia may be poorer following infiltration injections compared with that obtained with lidocaine and epinephrine.

Ropivacaine
Ropivacaine is similar to bupivacaine and has the same indications for use - namely, when long-lasting anaesthesia is required. Like bupivacaine it has to be drawn up from vials. The advantage over bupivacaine is that ropivacaine is less cardiotoxic. It is available in a number of formulations. Concentrations of 0.5% (with and without epinephrine), 0.75% and 1% have been used in dentistry. Like levobupivacaine, ropivacaine is presented as a single isomer, not a racemic mixture.

When used in medical practice the efficacy of ropivacaine has been reported to be equally effective with and without epinephrine. In dentistry the addition of epinephrine increases the duration of anaesthesia produced by ropivacaine.

Ester Local Anaesthetics
The ester local anaesthetics that may be used in dentistry are:
• procaine
• benzocaine
• amethocaine
• cocaine.

Only procaine is used as an injectable agent, the others may be used topically.

Procaine
Procaine was the first-choice local anaesthetic for dentistry until the advent of lidocaine. Unfortunately, procaine is no longer supplied in dental cartridges and if it is needed then it must be drawn up from an ampoule. The only indication for its use is in a patient allergic to all of the amide anaesthetics. This is extremely rare and it is unlikely that most practitioners will encounter this particular indication. In dentistry it is used as a 2% solution with epinephrine. Plain procaine is an excellent vasodilator. Therefore it may be used as an emergency intra-arterial drug to counter arteriospasm, which is a rare complication of intravenous sedation.

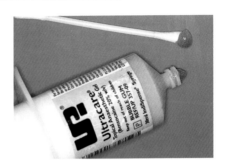

Fig 3-5 Benzocaine is only used as a topical anaesthetic.

Benzocaine
Benzocaine is used as a topical anaesthetic in dentistry. It cannot be injected, as this drug is insoluble in water. It is applied as a 20% gel when used as a topical agent (Fig 3-5).

Amethocaine
Amethocaine is not administered by injection as it has unacceptable toxicity. It is supplied as a 4% topical preparation for skin that may be used prior to venepuncture for intravenous sedation or general anaesthesia.

Cocaine
Cocaine is not employed much in dentistry these days due to its potential for misuse as an illicit substance. It is occasionally used as a topical anaesthetic. In this form it is applied as a solution in concentrations up to 10%.

Vasoconstrictors

Only two vasoconstrictors are used in dental local anaesthetic solutions marketed in the UK. They are:
- epinephrine
- felypressin.

Epinephrine
Epinephrine is a naturally occurring hormone. When added to dental local anaesthetic solutions it offers a number of advantages including
- more profound anaesthesia
- longer-lasting pulpal anaesthesia
- haemorrhage control.

In local anaesthetic solutions used in the UK the concentration of epinephrine varies from 1:80,000 (12.5 µg/mL) to 1:200,000 (5 µg/mL).

As it is a naturally occurring hormone, epinephrine has a number of effects. The unwanted effects and hazards of epinephrine are discussed in Chapter 7.

Felypressin

Felypressin is a synthetic octapeptide, which is very similar to the naturally occurring pituitary hormone vasopressin. It is added to dental local anaesthetic solutions in a concentration of 0.03 IU/mL (0.54µg/mL). Felypressin is not as profound a vasoconstrictor as epinephrine, so it is not as effective in haemorrhage control.

Which Local Anaesthetic Solutions Should I Have in My Surgery?

It is apparent from the above that there are a number of choices to be made in relation to the local anaesthetics that are available in the UK. This governs the anaesthetic solutions that should be kept in stock. The solutions in the dental clinic will vary from practice to practice depending upon the patient profile and the types of treatment offered. Having a number of different solutions in stock allows the provision of bespoke anaesthesia, which is

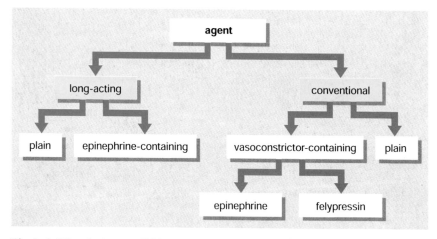

Fig 3-6 The choices available in relation to the type of local anaesthetic solution used.

the ideal. The decision-making process is summarised in diagrammatic form in Fig 3-6. Choice will be governed by the following factors:
• method of anaesthesia
• patient factors
• type of treatment.

Method of Anaesthesia

The various types of anaesthesia are described in the three chapters that follow and are shown in a flow diagram in Fig 3-7. When using conventional methods of dental anaesthesia pulpal anaesthesia is more profound when a vasoconstrictor-containing solution is used. Therefore vasoconstrictor-containing solutions are preferred. When using intraligamentary techniques it is essential to use an epinephrine-containing solution if acceptable levels of anaesthesia are to be achieved. Unless other influences override, the solution of choice for all the methods described is lidocaine with epinephrine.

Patient Factors

A number of factors related to the patient influence the choice of anaesthesia. Rare conditions include allergy to one of the amides indicating that another anaesthetic agent must be used. More commonly, the patient influ-

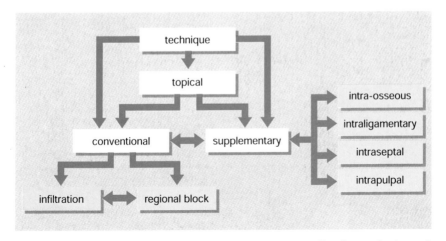

Fig 3-7 The choices available in relation to the technique of local anaesthesia used.

ences the choice concerning the vasoconstrictor. First, should a vasocon-strictor be avoided completely? Secondly, which vasoconstrictor is preferred? Situations in which vasoconstrictors are to be avoided are rare. The only time it may be encountered in dental practice is when anaesthetising a region that has been subjected to therapeutic irradiation for the treatment of malignan-cy. This treatment reduces the blood supply to the area and subsequent re-duction in blood supply produced by an injected vasoconstrictor, especial-ly during surgical treatments, can increase the chance of necrosis. In such circumstances plain mepivacaine or plain prilocaine solutions are the pre-ferred choice.

The more common dilemma is which of the two vasoconstrictors available should be chosen? Epinephrine is the preferred choice in most patients. Nev-ertheless, there are some indications for either dose-reduction or use of the alternative agent, felypressin. These indications are discussed more fully in Chapter 7. In brief, it is safer to use felypressin-containing solutions in pa-tients with severe cardiac disease, although this agent must also be used with care in these circumstances.

Type of Treatment

Periodontal and oral surgical treatments require good haemostasis. Epi-nephrine-containing solutions provide better haemorrhage control than those with felypressin. Thus the former are preferred for such procedures.

Long-acting local anaesthetics such as bupivacaine offer the possibility of prolonged pain relief after surgical procedures (Fig 3-8). Therefore these agents should be considered when regional block methods of anaesthesia are

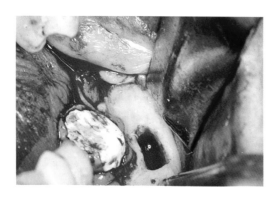

Fig 3-8 Long-acting local anaesthetics provide pro-longed pain relief following oral surgical procedures.

used during oral surgery. Operative pain control is better with lidocaine with epinephrine. However, the administration of bupivacaine will provide longer-lasting postoperative anaesthesia.

Conclusions

- A variety of local anaesthetics are supplied for use in dentistry.
- Epinephrine and felypressin are used as vasoconstrictors.
- The selection available allows bespoke anaesthesia.

Further Reading

Danielsson K, Evers H, Holmlund A, Kjellman O, Nordenram A, Personn N-E. Long-acting local anaesthetics in oral surgery. Int J Oral and Maxillofac Surg 1986;15:119-126.

Kennedy M, Reader A, Beck M, Weaver J. Anesthetic efficacy of ropivacaine in maxillary anterior infiltration. Oral Surg Oral Med Oral Path 2001;91:406-412.

Jastak JT, Yagiela JA, Donaldson D. Local Anesthesia of the Oral Cavity. Philadelphia: Saunders, 1995.

Chapter 4
Techniques for Maxillary Anaesthesia

Aim

The aim of this chapter is to describe the different methods available to anaesthetise the upper teeth and their associated structures.

Outcome

After reading this chapter you should have an understanding of the different local anaesthetic techniques used in the upper jaw. You will understand the indications for use of each method.

Introduction and Terminology

The maxillary teeth may be anaesthetised by infiltration, regional block, intraligamentary, intra-osseous and intrapulpal anaesthesia. The primary method is infiltration anaesthesia. This chapter will describe the infiltration and regional block methods used in the upper jaw.

As a general rule for all injections in both jaws the patient position should be such that it allows access to the point of injection while affording the safest and most comfortable placement for the patient. Ideally the patient should be fully supine to aid cranial blood flow and prevent fainting. Some patients may be uncomfortable or feel vulnerable in this position. A compromise is to tilt the chair back at least thirty degrees to the vertical.

Buccal Infiltration Anaesthesia

Solution deposited at the buccal side of the maxillary alveolus can infiltrate through to the pulps of the teeth to produce dental anaesthesia (Fig 4-1). This is because the cortical plate on the buccal side of the maxilla is thin. The advantages of infiltration anaesthesia are:
- simple technique which is easy to master
- when successful, anaesthetises all nerve endings in the area of deposition independent of the nerve source.

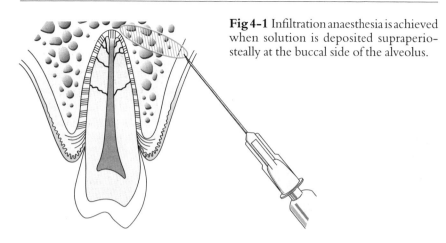

Fig 4-1 Infiltration anaesthesia is achieved when solution is deposited supraperiosteally at the buccal side of the alveolus.

The disadvantages are:
- only effective in obtaining pulpal anaesthesia when diffusion through cortical bone occurs
- localised infection may be spread if an inflamed area is infiltrated
- only a limited zone of anaesthesia per injection.

Technique
The syringe is fitted with a 27 or 30 gauge needle. Usually a 20-25 mm-long needle is employed. Unless there is a medical contraindication a vasoconstrictor-containing anaesthetic such as lidocaine with epinephrine is used.

The point of needle penetration is in the buccal fold within reflected mucosa (Fig 4-2). Access to this region is easiest when the patient has the mouth only partly open. This is especially the case in the more posterior regions of the buccal sulcus. When the mouth is fully open the buccal tissues are stretched across the teeth, limiting access. Prior to injection this area should be cleaned with a gauze swab and a topical anaesthetic applied. The operator pulls the cheek or lip in a superior direction to stretch the tissues and the needle is inserted through the taut tissues of the buccal fold. This stretching of the lip or cheek may be performed by holding the tissues between the operator's fingers (Fig 4-2) or by retraction with a mirror (Fig 4-3). The former method affords more control; the latter reduces the chances of needle-stick injury. The choice is personal. It is important to stretch the tissue at the puncture-point. This enables smooth needle penetration with minimal dragging of the mucosa. The needle must be inserted into a plane deeper

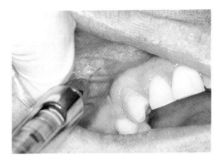

Fig 4-2 A maxillary buccal infiltration injection; access is achieved by pulling on the lip with the fingers.

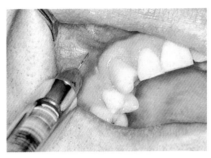

Fig 4-3 In this delivery of an infiltration injection, the lips are retracted by a dental mirror. This reduces the chances of a needlestick injury during the injection.

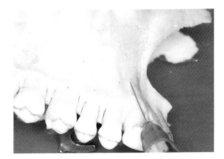

Fig 4-4 The position of the needle for an infiltration in the upper canine region.

than the epithelium. Injecting into the epithelium produces a distinct blister. This produces discomfort and, if noted, the needle is advanced to a deeper level. The needle is directed towards the bone, aiming for the apical area of the tooth in question (Fig 4-4). Bone does not need to be contacted. If bone is touched the needle should be withdrawn slightly so that the point is not subperiosteal. An injection underneath the periosteum is painful at the time and in the postanaesthetic stage. Before injecting, aspiration is performed. The incidence of positive aspiration during buccal anaesthesia is low (around 1-2%). If aspiration is negative then 1 mL of solution is deposited over a period of 30 seconds. At least two minutes should elapse before testing for the effect of the anaesthetic.

This technique will normally anaesthetise the pulps of the tooth in question and the contiguous teeth. The soft tissues on the buccal side, including the periodontal ligament and the buccal alveolar bone in the region, will also be anaesthetised.

Pulpal anaesthesia of around 45 minutes should ensue when a vasoconstrictor-containing solution has been used. The efficacy of infiltration anaesthesia is dependent upon the volume and concentration of the local anaesthetic solution and the presence of a vasoconstrictor. The efficacy of lidocaine as an anaesthetic during infiltration anaesthesia increases with increasing epinephrine concentration. Long-lasting local anaesthetics do not provide prolonged postoperative pain relief if injected by infiltration although soft tissue anaesthesia is prolonged.

Problems with buccal infiltration anaesthesia
Buccal infiltrations may fail if there is collateral supply to the pulp from the greater palatine or nasopalatine nerves. This is overcome by supplementing the injection with one of the palatal techniques described below.

Another reason for failure may be due to a thick cortical plate reducing the spread of solution through bone. This may occur in the region of the zygomatic buttress causing failure of anaesthesia in upper first molars. This is overcome by infiltrating mesially and distally to the buttress or by using the regional block methods described below. It must be remembered that the upper first molar tooth can receive supply from both the posterior and the middle superior alveolar nerves, thus two blocks may be required in some cases.

If there is localised infection at the site of an infiltration it is unwise to inject at this zone. Using one of the regional block methods described below surmounts this problem.

Palatal Infiltration

When working on the tissues distal to the canine the palatal soft tissue can be anaesthetised by infiltration (Fig 4-5) or regional block anaesthesia (see below). Infiltration of around 0.2 mL of solution into the palatal mucosa just distal to the tooth of interest will anaesthetise the palatal mucosa and periodontium anterior to the point of infiltration up to the canine region. The exception is the upper third molar when the solution should be deposited at the anterior aspect of the tooth. This is because the greater palatine foramen lies anterior to the third molar tooth (Fig 4-6) and the nerve supplying

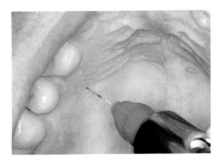 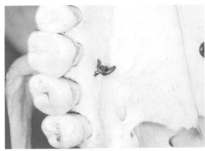

Fig 4-5 A palatal infiltration injection.

Fig 4-6 The position of the greater palatine foramen. It is anterior to the third molar.

this region travels in a posterior direction. The point of infiltration is in the fleshiest part of the palate around 10 to 15 mm from the gingival margin (Fig 4-5). The duration of infiltration and greater palatine nerve block anaesthesia in the palate is similar. Thus the choice of technique in the posterior part of the palate is personal. In the anterior region a nasopalatine block is the preferred method.

Palatal injections can be uncomfortable owing to the poor compliance of the tissue. Chapter 9 describes methods of reducing this discomfort by chasing local anaesthetic solution through from already anaesthetised buccal papillae.

Regional block methods in the maxilla
Regional block anaesthesia may be used in the maxilla if infiltration methods are ineffective or to avoid multiple injections when a large area of anaesthesia is needed. Only intraoral approaches will be described. It is possible to approach the maxillary nerve and some of its branches from extraoral approaches but these are not recommended in dental practice.

Regional block methods useful in the maxilla include:
• posterior superior alveolar nerve block
• maxillary molar nerve block
• middle superior alveolar nerve block
• anterior superior alveolar nerve block
• infraorbital nerve block
• palatal anterior superior alveolar nerve block

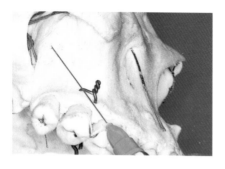

Fig 4-7 The position of the needle during a posterior superior alveolar nerve block.

- anterior middle superior alveolar nerve block
- greater palatine nerve block
- nasopalatine (long sphenopalatine nerve) block
- maxillary nerve block.

Posterior superior alveolar nerve block

The posterior superior alveolar nerve block supplies the pulps of the upper molar teeth with the possible exception of the mesiobuccal pulp of the upper first permanent molar, which receives innervation from the middle superior alveolar nerve when the latter is present. Depositing solution behind the maxillary tuberosity can block this nerve (Fig 4-7). The choice of needle length for this injection is governed by operator preference. Some operators use a short (25 mm) needle whereas others prefer the long (35 mm) version. The method is as follows. The patient has the mouth opened slightly and the buccal tissues are retracted. The needle is inserted at the height of the buccal sulcus in the plane of the distal surface of the second molar and advanced

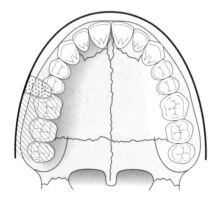

Fig 4-8 The extent of anaesthesia following a successful posterior superior alveolar nerve block The striped area shows complete anaesthesia, the stippled area partial anaesthesia.

close to the bony surface at an angle of 45° superiorly, posteriorly and medially to a depth of around 20 mm. At this point the tip of the needle is lying adjacent to the posterior wall of the maxillary tuberosity. Aspiration is performed and 1-1.5 mL of solution deposited. The zone of anaesthesia is illustrated in Fig 4-8.

Haematoma formation may be an undesirable side effect of this technique. If this happens, firm pressure must be applied in the pterygoid region for a minimum of 5 minutes. Limitation of mouth opening can affect the patient for up to two weeks if a haematoma is formed.

Maxillary molar nerve block

This technique is a modification of the posterior superior alveolar nerve block. This method was developed to overcome failure of anaesthesia in the maxillary first molar owing to accessory supply from the middle superior alveolar nerve, as this nerve may supply the mesiobuccal pulp of the first molar. In addition, it is claimed that this technique does not produce the same incidence of haematoma formation, which may be associated with posterior superior alveolar nerve blocks. The method is as follows. The patient has the mouth half-closed and the zygomatic process of the maxilla is located with a finger. The finger is advanced distally towards the maxillary tuberosity (Figs 4-9a,b). The needle is inserted high in the buccal sulcus between the finger and the distal surface of the zygomatic process. The needle is advanced around 10 mm into the space above the buccinator attachment. Following aspiration at this site about 2 mL of local anaesthetic solution is injected while maintaining finger pressure. A swelling is produced

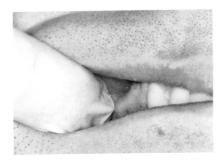

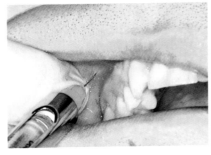

Fig 4-9a Palpating the zygomatic process and advancing the finger to the tuberosity prior to a maxillary molar nerve block.

Fig 4-9b Delivering the maxillary molar nerve block.

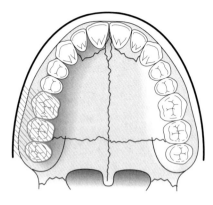

Fig 4-10 The extent of anaesthesia following a successful maxillary molar nerve block.

above buccinator as the solution is injected. Once the needle is withdrawn the patient is asked to close the mouth slightly and a finger massages the solution superiorly, medially and distally towards the posterior superior alveolar foramen. The region anaesthetised is illustrated in Fig 4-10.

Middle superior alveolar nerve block

The middle superior alveolar nerve provides innervation to the premolar pulps as well as the mesiobuccal pulp of the maxillary first permanent molar tooth. The administration of an infraorbital nerve block (see below) will often suffice to block the middle superior alveolar nerve except in those circumstances where the nerve leaves the infraorbital nerve in a posterior part of the infraorbital canal. In the latter case a middle superior dental nerve block can be used. This is achieved by inserting the needle in the buccal sulcus in the second premolar region. The needle is advanced to a supraperiosteal position close to the apex of the second premolar tooth and 1.5 mL

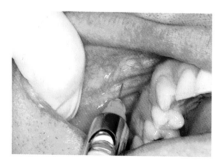

Fig 4-11 A middle superior alveolar nerve block.

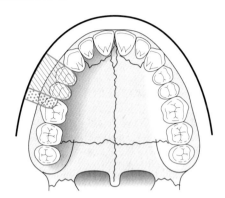

Fig 4-12 The extent of anaesthesia following a successful middle superior alveolar nerve block. The striped area shows complete anaesthesia, the stippled area partial anaesthesia.

of solution deposited (Fig 4-11). The extent of anaesthesia is illustrated in Fig 4-12.

Anterior superior alveolar nerve block

The anterior superior alveolar nerve supplies the canine and upper incisor teeth. There is some crossover at the midline from the contralateral supply. The anterior superior alveolar nerve may be blocked in isolation or by the infraorbital nerve block described below. The former technique is performed by introducing the needle into the buccal sulcus in the maxillary canine region and advancing the needle towards the canine apex. The needle is maintained in a supraperiosteal position and following aspiration 1.5 mL of solution is deposited. The zone of anaesthesia is illustrated in Fig 4-13.

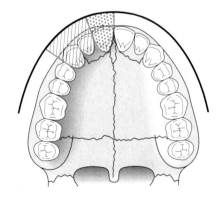

Fig 4-13 The extent of anaesthesia following a successful anterior superior alveolar nerve block. The striped area shows complete anaesthesia, the stippled area partial anaesthesia.

47

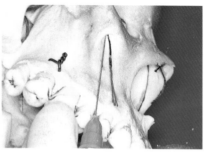

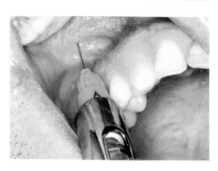

Fig 4-14 Position of the needle during an infraorbital nerve block.

Fig 4-15 An infraorbital nerve block.

Infraorbital nerve block

The infraorbital nerve block (Fig 4-14) produces anaesthesia of one side of the upper lip and part of the skin of the nose. The intraoral approach is as follows. The patient has the mouth open slightly and the tissues are retracted laterally. A long (35 mm) needle should be used. The needle pierces the height of the buccal sulcus in the mid-premolar region (Fig 4-15). It is advanced superiorly parallel to the premolar roots until bony contact is made in the region of the infraorbital foramen that is being palpated extraorally by the index finger. The needle is then withdrawn slightly to a supraperiosteal position. Aspiration is performed and 1 mL of solution should be injected slowly.

The infraorbital nerve block will anaesthetise the anterior superior alveolar nerve on one side. This nerve leaves the trunk of the infraorbital nerve about

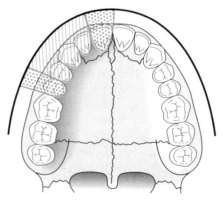

Fig 4-16 The extent of anaesthesia following a successful infraorbital nerve block. The striped area shows complete anaesthesia, the stippled area partial anaesthesia.

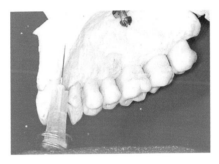 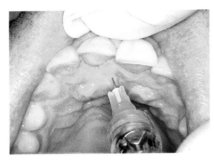

Fig 4-17 Position of the needle during a palatal anterior superior alveolar nerve block.

Fig 4-18 A palatal anterior superior alveolar nerve block.

5 mm before the foramen to supply the pulps of the anterior maxillary teeth on one side. In the absence of a middle superior alveolar nerve it also innervates the premolar teeth. The zone of anaesthesia is illustrated in Fig 4-16.

Palatal anterior superior alveolar nerve block

This is a means of anaesthetising the upper anterior teeth (canine to canine and sometimes the premolars as well) by depositing solution deep in the incisive canal (Fig 4-17). The solution gains entry to the cancellous bone of the maxilla via the canal and from here reaches the pulps of the teeth. This method relies on the very slow delivery of local anaesthetic using a computerised delivery system. The use of computerised delivery systems reduces injection discomfort and patient anxiety. The method is reputed to provide pulpal anaesthesia of the maxillary anterior teeth bilaterally without loss of sensation labially. Unlike the methods described earlier it is essential to have the patient open the mouth wide for this technique. The needle is inserted slowly into the incisive papilla (Fig 4-18). Controlling a drop of solution on the point of the needle and placing the bevel against the mucosa to press the solution into the mucosa may help reduce the discomfort of penetration. The needle is then advanced into the incisive foramen and advanced along its length maintaining injection throughout. Around 1 mL of solution is deposited deep into the canal.

Anterior middle superior alveolar nerve block

Like the palatal anterior superior block this technique relies on the use of a computerised delivery system and is claimed to provide pulpal anaesthesia without facial numbness. It is a palatal approach to both the anterior and

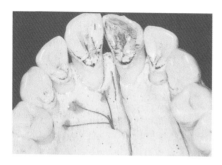

Fig 4-19 The palatal cortex contains a number of bony perforations that permit entry of local anaesthetic solution into the cancellous bone.

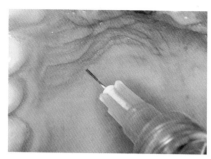

Fig 4-20 An anterior middle superior alveolar nerve block.

middle superior alveolar nerves. Although the palatal cortex is thick it contains a number of perforations that permit entry of solution into the cancellous part of the maxilla (Fig 4-19). The patient has the mouth opened wide and the point of injection is midway between the gingival margin and the midline of the palate between the first and second premolars (Fig 4-20). Around 1 mL of solution is deposited slowly at this site and it is claimed that this will produce anaesthesia of the teeth on that side from the central incisor to the second premolar, although crossover supply at the midline would be expected to be problematic in the central incisor region. It has been suggested that excessive blanching of the tissues during injection with this method can lead to ulceration of the palatal mucosa.

Greater palatine nerve block

As mentioned above, it is possible to anaesthetise the palatal tissues by infiltration or by regional block methods. The greater palatine nerve block anaesthetises the soft tissues of the hard palate from third molar to canine region. The greater palatine foramen is located palatally to the distal aspect of the upper second molar tooth. The use of a ball-ended instrument such as an amalgam condenser is useful in locating the site of this foramen (Fig 4-21). This is the site of anaesthetic deposition (Fig 4-22). The needle is inserted only a few millimetres and aspiration performed. Very little anaesthetic solution is required to obtain a greater palatine nerve block. Around 0.2 mL is sufficient.

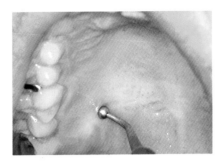

Fig 4-21 A round-ended instrument such as an amalgam condenser is useful in locating the greater palatine foramen.

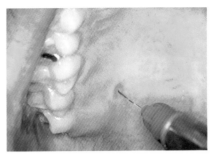

Fig 4-22 A greater palatine nerve block.

Fig 4-23 The area anaesthetised by a greater palatine nerve block. The striped area shows complete anaesthesia, the stippled area partial anaesthesia.

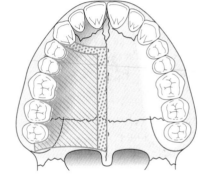

This injection anaesthetises the soft tissues and bone of the hard palate on one side of the midline up to the canine region (Fig 4-23). Some fibres from the nasopalatine nerve, however, may encroach upon the canine region.

Nasopalatine (long sphenopalatine nerve) block
This injection anaesthetises the soft tissues of the anterior hard palate in the incisor region bilaterally. There is some crossover supply in the canine region from the greater palatine nerve. During the injection the patient has the mouth wide open. The needle is inserted at one side of the incisive papilla (Fig 4-24). Penetration of only a few millimetres is required; aspiration is performed and less than 0.2 mL of solution deposited. Anaesthesia occurs rapidly following this injection.

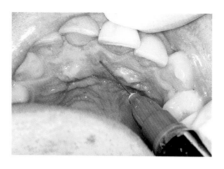

Fig 4-24 A nasopalatine nerve block.

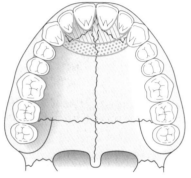

Fig 4-25 The extent of anaesthesia following a successful nasopalatine nerve block. The striped area shows complete anaesthesia, the stippled area partial anaesthesia.

This injection anaesthetises the soft tissues and bone of the anterior hard palate adjacent to the six anterior teeth (Fig 4-25). In the canine region some fibres from the greater palatine nerve may provide an accessory supply.

In order to reduce the discomfort of this injection the incisive papilla may be approached via previously anaesthetised buccal tissues by chasing the anaesthetic through the central incisor interdental papilla.

Maxillary nerve block
There are two approaches to the maxillary nerve block – namely, the tuberosity approach and the greater palatine canal approach (Figs 4-26a,b). The former is similar to the posterior superior alveolar nerve block, the latter gains access to the maxillary nerve trunk via the greater palatine canal. Deposition of local anaesthetic solution around the trunk of the maxillary nerve will provide anaesthesia of one-half of the upper jaw, including all of the teeth and the buccal and palatal mucosa (Fig 4-27).

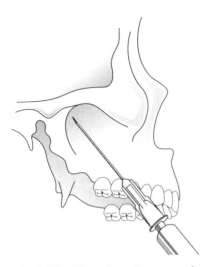

Fig 4-26a The tuberosity approach to the maxillary nerve block.

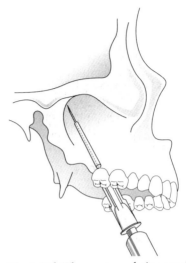

Fig 4-26b The greater palatine canal approach to the maxillary nerve block.

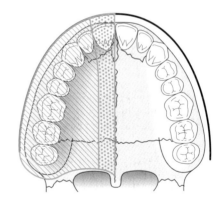

Fig 4-27 The extent of anaesthesia following a successful maxillary nerve block. The striped area shows complete anaesthesia, the stippled area partial anaesthesia.

Tuberosity approach

A long (35 mm) needle must be used. The approach is identical to the posterior superior alveolar nerve block (Fig 4-7). However, the needle is inserted to a much greater depth - namely, 30 mm. At this point the needle is in the vicinity of the maxillary nerve within the pterygopalatine fossa. This end point is superior and medial to the point of injection during the posterior superior alveolar nerve block. Following aspiration, 2 mL of solution is injected. There is a high risk of haematoma with this injection.

53

Greater palatine canal approach

The patient has the mouth open wide and the greater palatine foramen is approached from the opposite side. The needle is advanced into the canal superiorly and posteriorly at an angle of 45°. The needle is advanced very slowly along the canal to a depth of 30 mm and 2 mL of solution deposited. If bony obstructions are encountered, the needle should not be advanced forcibly. It is better to withdraw slightly and advance again at a different angle. If an insurmountable barrier is encountered then this approach should be abandoned. Bleeding at the needle exit point can occur with this injection. Firm pressure at the site for a few minutes will arrest any haemorrhage.

Conclusions

- Infiltration and regional block anaesthesia may be used in the maxilla.
- The usual method is infiltration anaesthesia.
- Regional block methods may be used if infiltration is ineffective or if extensive areas of anaesthesia are required.
- Computerised delivery systems have allowed novel methods of regional block anaesthesia.

Further Reading

Adatia AK. Regional nerve block for maxillary permanent molars. Br Dent J 1976;140:87-92.

Friedman MJ, Hochman MN. P-ASA block injection: A new palatal technique to anesthetize maxillary anterior teeth. J Esthetic Dent 1999;11:63-71.

Friedman MJ, Hochman MN. The AMSA injection: A new concept for local anesthesia of maxillary teeth using a computer-controlled injection system. Quintessence Int 1998;29:297-303.

Chapter 5
Techniques for Mandibular Anaesthesia

Aim

The aim of this chapter is to describe the different methods available to anaesthetise the lower teeth and their associated structures.

Outcome

After reading this chapter you should have an understanding of the different local anaesthetic techniques used in the lower jaw. You will understand the indications for use of each method.

Introduction and Terminology

Unlike the maxilla, where infiltration is the normal method, in the mandible both infiltration and regional block techniques may be considered as first-choice injections. The decision as to which to use is governed by:
• the age of the patient
• the tooth of interest.

It was mentioned in Chapter 4 that the patient position should allow access to the point of injection while affording the safest and most comfortable placement for the patient. The fully supine position aids cranial blood flow and prevents fainting but some patients may be uncomfortable or feel vulnerable in this position. A compromise position of tilting the chair back at least thirty degrees to the vertical is suggested. In some mandibular block techniques this tilted position provides an additional advantage. This is because when the mouth is wide open the mandibular occlusal plane is almost horizontal. This is useful in locating the appropriate landmarks.

Infiltration Methods

Age of the patient
Infiltration anaesthesia is the method of choice for anaesthesia of the deciduous dentition in children. The technique is similar to that described for

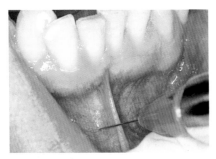

Fig 5-1 Buccal infiltration anaesthesia may be effective in the mandibular anterior region in adults.

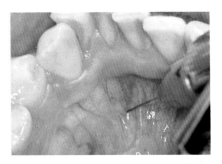

Fig 5-2 Lingual infiltration when combined with buccal infiltration can provide reliable pulpal anaesthesia in anterior mandibular teeth in adults.

maxillary buccal infiltrations as the approach is from the buccal side. In the lower jaw the area of penetration is made taut by pulling the tissues laterally and inferiorly rather than superiorly. The point of penetration is in the depth of the buccal sulcus and the technique is identical to maxillary buccal infiltration as described in Chapter 4. A 30-gauge needle is used and 1 mL of solution deposited over 30 seconds.

Tooth of interest

In adults, infiltration anaesthesia is the first choice for pulpal anaesthesia of the lower incisor teeth. Regional block injections are poor in this regard, partly due to supply from the contralateral inferior alveolar nerve. Pulpal anaesthesia is best achieved by depositing solution both buccally and lingually in the apical region of the tooth involved. A volume of at least 0.5 mL at each site is recommended. The buccal injection is as described above (Fig 5-1). The lingual infiltration is performed in the reflected mucosa in the apical region of the tooth of interest (Fig 5-2). The onset of anaesthesia may take longer than a maxillary buccal infiltration. It may be 8 to 10 minutes before pulpal anaesthesia is of sufficient depth to allow pain-free operative procedures on the tooth.

Regional Block Methods

Most dental treatment on the adult dentition that requires anaesthesia is performed using regional block methods. In Chapter 4 the advantages and disadvantages of infiltration anaesthesia were listed. The advantages of regional block techniques are:

- they produce widespread anaesthesia from one injection
- the anaesthetic can be deposited away from infected areas.

The disadvantages of block injections are:
- they are technically more difficult than infiltration anaesthesia
- they do not anaesthetise nerve endings from different trunks (for example, in the mid-line where crossover may occur).
- they produce excessive soft tissue anaesthesia
- they may cause deep haemorrhage in patients with bleeding diatheses
- although rare, the potential for direct injury to a nerve trunk is possible.

Regional block methods in the mandible

As is the case with the maxilla, there are extraoral approaches to the mandibular nerve. These are not recommended in dental practice and only intraoral techniques will be described. Regional block methods used in the mandible include:
- inferior alveolar and lingual nerve block
- Gow-Gates block
- Akinosi-Vazirani block
- incisive and mental nerve block
- long buccal nerve block
- mylohyoid nerve block.

The inferior alveolar and lingual nerve block

The inferior alveolar nerve block is probably the method used by most practitioners for anaesthesia in the adult mandible. The aim of the injection is to deposit local anaesthetic solution close to the mandibular foramen on the

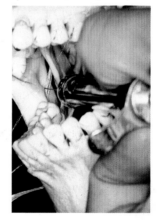

Fig 5-3 Deposition of local anaesthetic solution at the mandibular foramen can block the inferior alveolar nerve.

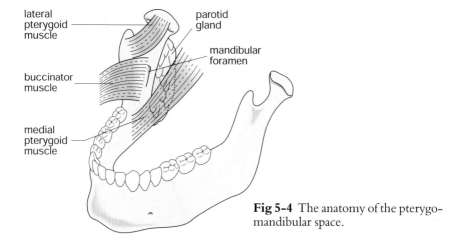

lateral pterygoid muscle

parotid gland

mandibular foramen

buccinator muscle

medial pterygoid muscle

Fig 5-4 The anatomy of the pterygo-mandibular space.

medial aspect of the mandibular ramus thus blocking transmission in the inferior alveolar nerve at the point of entry into the bone (Fig 5-3). There are a number of approaches to the mandibular foramen.

1. The direct technique
This method is also known as the Halstead approach and relies on simple anatomical landmarks. The aim is to deposit the local anaesthetic in the pterygomandibular space. This anatomical space is bordered posteriorly by the parotid gland, laterally by the ramus of the mandible, medially and inferiorly by the medial pterygoid muscle, superiorly by the lateral pterygoid muscle and anteriorly by the buccinator muscle (Fig 5-4). As the object is to deposit solution close to the mandibular foramen, the dentist should use all the

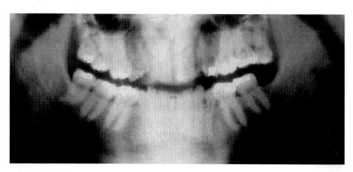

Fig 5-5 A panoramic radiograph can help in localising the mandibular foramina.

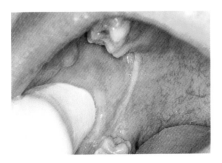

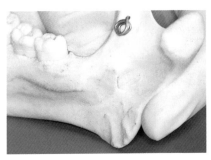

Fig 5-6 The operator's thumb locates the coronoid notch of the ramus of the mandible.

Fig 5-7 In adults the mandibular foramen is halfway between the operator's thumb and finger when the ramus is held as shown.

information that is available to help locate this target. The standard anatomical pointers are given below, but the position of the foramen is variable. It should be noted that the mandibular foramen is usually apparent on dental panoramic radiographs (Fig 5-5) and if one of these is available it should be consulted. Information regarding the height (in relation to the teeth) and anteroposterior position of the foramen will be obtained from the radiograph.

In adults a 27-gauge long needle is recommended. This is due to the depth of penetration that may be required; it is often around 25 mm. A needle should not be inserted to its hub (when using a short 25 mm needle this could occur). This is because it is at the hub at which needles fracture when stressed. This is a very rare occurrence. If a needle did fracture in the pterygomandibular space and there was nothing to grab hold of in the mouth a surgical procedure would be required for removal. Surgery in this site has the potential to produce nerve damage and is best avoided. This is why in most adults a long needle is recommended. The patient's mouth is opened wide and the ramus is held between the operator's thumb and index finger. The thumb is placed in the mandibular retromolar region in the coronoid notch of the ascending ramus (Fig 5-6). Before reaching this final resting point the thumb has stretched the mucosa over the ramus and in doing so achieves two important functions. First, the thumb has palpated the internal oblique ridge of the mandible and a mental note is made of its position. Secondly, this action has stretched the mucosa to enable easier needle penetration. The index or middle finger is placed extraorally on the posterior aspect of the ramus at the same height as the thumb. In the adult mandible the mandibular foramen is often approximately halfway between the oper-

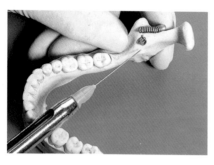

Fig 5-8 The direct approach to the mandibular foramen during an inferior alveolar nerve block.

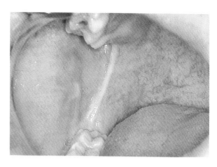

Fig 5-9 The pterygomandibular raphe appears as a pale band running in a vertical direction medial to the ramus.

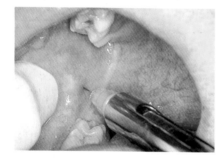

Fig 5-10 The direct or Halstead approach to the inferior alveolar nerve block.

ator's thumb and index finger about halfway up the thumbnail (Fig 5-7). The syringe is introduced across the premolars of the opposite side (Fig 5-8) aiming to enter mucosa at the level of halfway up the operator's thumbnail.

The point of entry is midway between the internal oblique ridge (which was palpated by the thumb) and the pterygomandibular raphe (which is visualised) (Fig 5-9). The needle is advanced through tissue until bony contact is made (Fig 5-10). In adults this normally occurs between 15 and 25 mm of penetration. If bony contact is made too soon then the area contacted is probably the internal oblique ridge of the mandible. Deposition of solution here will not anaesthetise the inferior alveolar nerve. If bone is not palpated then it is possible that the needle is placed too far posteriorly. This can result in the needle entering the parotid gland. Injection into this gland can produce loss of transmission in the motor fibres of the facial nerve (this is a

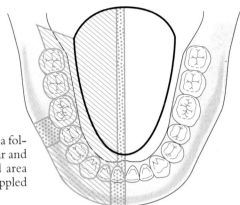

Fig 5-11 The extent of anaesthesia following a successful inferior alveolar and lingual nerve block. The striped area shows complete anaesthesia, the stippled area partial anaesthesia.

temporary but embarrassing problem and is discussed in Chapter 7). When the needle has contacted bone in the correct position it is withdrawn slightly, aspiration performed and 1.5 mL of solution deposited slowly. Aspiration is important, as positive aspirates in up to 20% of inferior alveolar injections using the direct method have been reported. This injection anaesthetises the inferior alveolar nerve and may block transmission in the lingual nerve. When lingual nerve anaesthesia is definitely required a modification to the technique is added. Following injection at the original site the needle is withdrawn halfway through mucosa, aspiration performed and solution deposited at this point. The injection continues as the needle is completely withdrawn, stopping just as the needle exits mucosa to prevent local anaesthetic spilling into the mouth. The extent of anaesthesia produced by the inferior alveolar and lingual nerve blocks is shown in Fig 5-11.

Success of the inferior alveolar nerve block is dependent upon the concentration of local anaesthetic but seems to be independent of the type of vaso-constrictor-containing solution employed. Similarly, the concentration of epinephrine (when present) does not appear to influence efficacy. Different teeth show different success rates: molars are more often successfully anaesthetised than incisors. Importantly, lip and tongue numbness are not a guarantee of pulpal anaesthesia. Reasons for failure with inferior alveolar nerve blocks are discussed below and in Chapter 8.

2. The indirect technique

This modification of the inferior alveolar nerve block is useful in overcoming the problem of contacting bone too soon with the direct method. As with the direct technique the patient has the mouth wide open and the op-

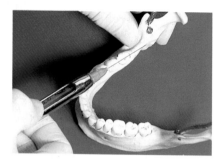

Fig 5-12 The initial position of the needle during the indirect approach to the inferior alveolar nerve block.

erator holds the patient's mandible in the manner described above. This time the needle is introduced across the occlusal plane of the mandibular teeth on the same side as the injection (Fig 5-12). The needle penetrates the same point in the mucosa as described above. After the needle has been inserted about a centimetre the syringe is swung across to the premolars of the opposite side and the injection then continues as described above for the direct method.

As this method involves more movement of the syringe than the direct technique, the latter method is preferred as first choice.

3. Anterior ramus technique

This method (known as the ART mandibular nerve block) was first described in 1997. The method relies on some of the landmarks used in the direct and indirect techniques. Owing to the amount of needle movement, the use of a broad-gauge needle (25 gauge) is advocated in the original description of the method. The operator's thumb palpates the coronoid notch on the anterior aspect of the ramus. The operator's middle or index finger palpates the distal surface of the mandible to assess the width of the ramus. A long (35 mm) needle is used. The needle is inserted buccally to the molars on the ipsilateral side to contact bone at the coronoid notch (Fig 5-13a), the needle is then advanced in a medial and posterior direction for half its length (Fig 5-13b). Once inserted to this depth the syringe is rotated about 30 degrees in the horizontal plane so that it rests over the anterior mandibular teeth on the ipsilateral side (Fig 5-13c). Following aspiration, the solution is administered at this point.

No data are reported relating to the success of this technique but the proponents of it claim that, as this method aims to deliver local anaesthetic in the lower aspect of the pterygomandibular space, it avoids the complications

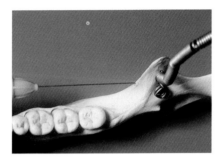

Fig 5-13a The initial position of the needle during the ART block.

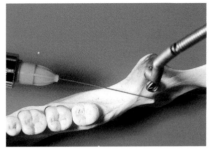

Fig 5-13b The intermediate position of the needle during the ART block.

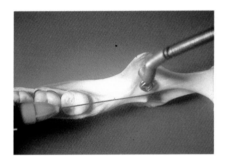

Fig 5-13c The final position of the needle during the ART block.

of "higher" techniques such as Akinosi-Vazirani and Gow-Gates (see below). Unwanted effects of these latter methods include entry into the maxillary or middle meningeal arteries and veins.

Problems with inferior alveolar nerve block anaesthesia
The inferior alveolar nerve block is not successful in 100% of cases. There are a number of reasons why an inferior alveolar nerve block may not be effective. These include:
i. Poor technique.
ii. An ectopic mandibular foramen. This foramen is not in the same position in every patient (and therefore the standard anatomical landmarks will not apply in every case). As mentioned above, panoramic radiographs may help localise the foramen. In addition, the position varies with age. In young patients the foramen may be below the occlusal plane, in adults it is usually above this level (Fig 5-14).
iii. Bending of the needle during administration. Dental local anaesthetic

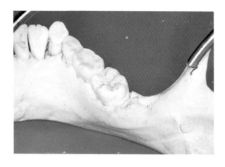

Fig 5-14 The mandibular foramen is below the occlusal plane in children.

needles are not rigid structures and may be deflected during advancement through tissues. Thus the needle may not reach the intended target area. It is possible that operators compensate for this and changing to different needles may lead to increased failure. Bending may be prevented by rotation of the needle during insertion. Such manipulation of the needle is possible with some computerised delivery systems but is difficult with a conventional syringe.

iv. Accessory nerve supply. The inferior alveolar nerve block may not provide satisfactory anaesthesia owing to the fact that nerves other than the inferior alveolar can provide innervation to the pulps of mandibular teeth. Among the nerves implicated as accessory suppliers are:
- the lingual nerve
- the long buccal nerve
- the mylohyoid nerve
- the auriculotemporal nerve
- the upper cervical nerves.

In addition, it should be remembered that those teeth close to the midline might receive bilateral innervation. As mentioned above, infiltration anaesthetic methods are recommended for the lower incisors.

The lingual nerve, of course, is often anaesthetised during the inferior alveolar nerve block and thus is not often a concern. The long buccal nerve may have to be anaesthetised by a separate injection if the standard inferior alveolar nerve block has been used. The long buccal nerve block is described below. The cervical supply may be countered by infiltration injections. Using "high" techniques such as the methods described below can block mylohyoid and auriculotemporal supply.

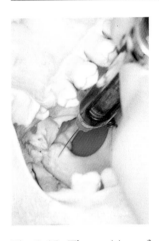

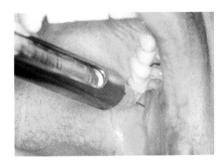

Fig 5-16 A Gow-Gates block.

Fig 5-15 The position of the needle during a Gow-Gates block.

Fig 5-17 The extent of anaesthesia following a successful Gow-Gates block. The striped area shows complete anaesthesia, the stippled area partial anaesthesia.

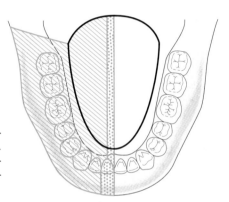

Gow-Gates mandibular nerve block

This method is one of the "high" methods of anaesthetising the inferior alveolar nerve. The aim is to deposit solution at the mandibular condyle (Fig 5-15). The advantage of this method is that it can block transmission in many accessory supplies to the dental pulps including that provided by the lingual, long buccal, mylohyoid and auriculotemporal nerves. The technique involves having the patient's mouth opened wide. The syringe is introduced into the mouth parallel to a plane running from the angle of the mouth to the inter-tragal notch of the ear across the opposite maxillary canine. The syringe is then directed across the palatal cusps of the maxillary second molar on the side receiving the injection and enters the mucosa at a point much higher than that penetrated during the standard Halstead approach (Fig 5-16). The needle is advanced through mucosa until bony contact is made on the condyle, withdrawn slightly and after aspiration the contents of the cartridge are deposited. The patient maintains the mouth in the open position

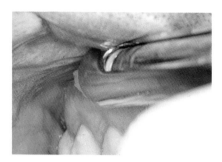

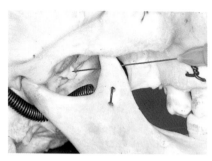

Fig 5-18 An Akinosi-Vazirani block.

Fig 5-19 Needle position during an Akinosi-Vazirani block.

for a few minutes. When initially described it was recommended that 3 mL of solution was used and thus a second injection may be required. The area anaesthetised is shown in Fig 5-17.

There is evidence that this technique is more successful than the conventional inferior alveolar nerve block and that there is less likelihood of intravascular injection.

Akinosi-Vazirani block

This is another "high" block. It is often referred to as the "Akinosi" technique. Uniquely for an intraoral approach to the inferior alveolar nerve it has no bony end-point and is administered with the patient's mouth closed. As was the case with the Gow-Gates technique, it may anaesthetise accessory supply to the dental pulps from the lingual, long buccal and mylohyoid nerves.

The technique is as follows. The patient has the mouth closed and the needle is introduced parallel to, and at the level of, the mucogingival junction along the maxillary alveolus on the side to be injected (Fig 5-18). A long 35 mm needle is used in adults. The needle is advanced posteriorly and enters mucosa high in the buccal sulcus. The needle is advanced until the hub is parallel to the distal surface of the second maxillary molar and at this point the solution is injected (Fig 5-19). The zone of anaesthesia is shown in Fig 5-20. The important landmarks for this technique are shown in Fig 5-21.

The success of the Akinosi method is variable. Some operators are more successful with the direct method whereas others are not. Advantages over the direct technique include less likelihood of intravascular injection and more

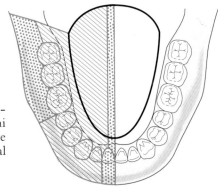

Fig 5-20 The extent of anaesthesia following a successful Akinosi-Vazirani block. The striped area shows complete anaesthesia, the stippled area partial anaesthesia.

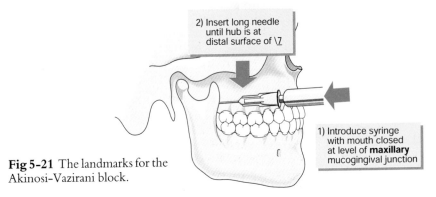

2) Insert long needle until hub is at distal surface of \7

1) Introduce syringe with mouth closed at level of **maxillary** mucogingival junction

Fig 5-21 The landmarks for the Akinosi-Vazirani block.

chance of anaesthetising accessory nerves. In addition, it can achieve anaesthesia of the inferior alveolar nerve in cases where access to the normal approach is difficult due to trismus or because of a large or uncontrollable tongue.

Incisive and mental nerve block

The incisive and mental nerve block involves depositing local anaesthetic solution at the mental foramen (Fig 5-22). The hope is that sufficient solution will enter the foramen to block transmission in the incisive nerve to anaesthetise the premolar and anterior mandibular teeth. As is the case with the mandibular foramen, the mental foramen is not in a constant position although it can be visualised in periapical radiographs. Unfortunately, it is not always apparent on panoramic radiographs. This injection is useful in providing soft tissue anaesthesia, as the mental nerve is readily accessible in the soft tissues. The amount entering the foramen to anaesthetise the inci-

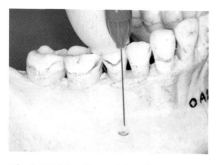

Fig 5-22 Needle position during an incisive and mental nerve block.

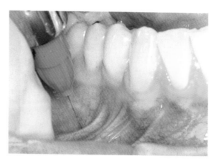

Fig 5-23 An incisive and mental nerve block injection.

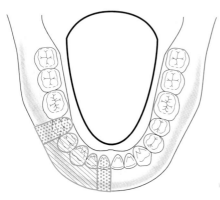

Fig 5-24 The extent of anaesthesia following a successful incisive and mental nerve block. The striped area shows complete anaesthesia, the stippled area partial anaesthesia.

sive branch must vary. The method is similar to that described for buccal infiltrations. The patient has the mouth partly open and the needle is inserted through reflected mucosa aiming for bone in the region between the premolar apices (Fig 5-23). Once bone is contacted the needle is withdrawn slightly, aspiration performed and 1.5 mL of solution deposited slowly. Massaging the tissues following injection may encourage entry of solution into the mental foramen. Pulpal anaesthesia is not as reliable following incisive nerve blocks compared with inferior alveolar nerve blocks. Incisive nerve block anaesthesia is unreliable for lower incisors but premolar pulpal anaesthesia of short duration can be obtained. The extent of anaesthesia is illustrated in Fig 5-24.

Long buccal nerve anaesthesia
The long buccal nerve may be anaesthetised at various points along its length.

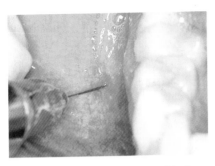

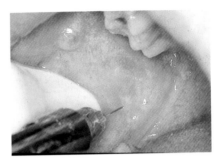

Fig 5-25 Anaesthetising part of the long buccal nerve by injection in reflected mucosa distal to the tooth of interest.

Fig 5-26 A long buccal nerve block.

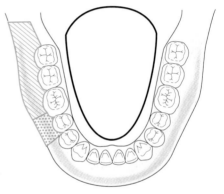

Fig 5-27 The extent of anaesthesia following a successful long buccal nerve block. The striped area shows complete anaesthesia, the stippled area partial anaesthesia.

Transmission in this nerve can be affected by depositing solution in the buccal tissues just distal to the tooth of interest (Fig 5-25). This may be performed in a zone from the depth of the mandibular buccal sulcus to the occlusal plane level in the buccal mucosa. Alternatively, a true long buccal block can be performed by depositing solution at the anterior aspect of the mandibular ramus (Fig 5-26). The coronoid notch is palpated as described above for the inferior alveolar nerve block and the needle is inserted at this point until bony contact is made. The needle is withdrawn slightly, aspiration performed and 0.5 mL of solution injected slowly. The area anaesthetised by a long buccal block is illustrated in Fig 5-27. The true block injection is preferred if accessory supply from this nerve enters the mandible distal to the last standing tooth. In some patients an anastomosis exists between the long buccal nerve and the inferior alveolar nerve and the former nerve may send accessory supply to the pulps of the teeth via retromolar foramina (see Chapter 8).

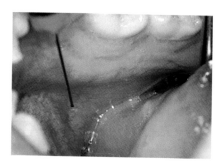 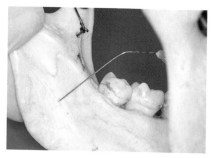

Fig 5-28a A mylohyoid nerve block.

Fig 5-28b An alternative method of anaesthetising the mylohyoid nerve at the mylohyoid groove.

Mylohyoid nerve block

The mylohyoid nerve is recognised as a source of accessory nerve supply to the pulps of the mandibular dentition, especially the anterior teeth. As this nerve leaves the inferior alveolar nerve over a centimetre above the mandibular foramen it may not be blocked by the standard approach to the inferior alveolar nerve leading to failure of pulpal anaesthesia. It is anaesthetised by the "high" techniques such as the Gow-Gates and the Akinosi methods. The nerve can also be anaesthetised by a mylohyoid nerve block (Figs 5-28a,b). The patient has the mouth opened widely and the tongue is reflected by a dental mirror. This injection deposits solution beneath the mylohyoid muscle in the region of the distal root of the first molar tooth (Fig 5-28a). An alternative method that deposits solution at the mylohyoid groove about a centimetre anterior to the mandibular foramen on the medial aspect of the mandible is also described. This method uses a long 27-gauge needle with a 107° bend in the shaft. The syringe is advanced across the occlusal plane of the mandibular incisors and the bent needle is inserted lingually to the retromolar fossa and inserted to a depth of 15 mm where it approximates the mylohyoid groove (Fig 5-28b). As a general rule, the use of bent needles is not recommended; thus the former method is preferred.

The mylohyoid nerve block when used alone does not provide reliable anaesthesia of the mandibular teeth.

Conclusions

- Infiltration and regional block anaesthesia are used in the mandible.
- Infiltration is the method of choice for the deciduous dentition.
- Infiltration is the method of choice for the lower incisors.
- A variety of methods of anaesthetising the inferior alveolar nerve are available.

Further Reading

Afsar A, Haas DA, Rossouw PE, Wood RE. Radiographic localization of mandibular anesthesia landmarks. Oral Surg Oral Med Oral Path 1998;86:234-241.

Akinosi JO. A new approach to the mandibular nerve block. Br J Oral Surg 1977;15:83-87.

Clark S, Reader A, Beck M, Meyers WJ. Anesthetic efficacy of the mylohyoid nerve block and combination inferior alveolar nerve/mylohyoid nerve block. Oral Surg Oral Med Oral Path 1999;87:557-563.

Chapter 6
Supplementary Techniques

Aim

The aim of this chapter is to describe methods of anaesthesia other than infiltration and regional block methods that are used in dentistry.

Outcome

After reading this chapter you should have an understanding of the usefulness and indications for supplementary anaesthetic techniques in the mouth.

Introduction and Terminology

The methods of anaesthesia described in this chapter are:
• topical anaesthesia
• jet injection
• intrapapillary anaesthesia
• intraosseous anaesthesia
• intraligamentary anaesthesia
• intraseptal anaesthesia
• intrapulpal anaesthesia
• transcutaneous electronic nerve stimulation.

All of these techniques can be used in either jaw.

Topical Anaesthesia

Topical anaesthetics may achieve beneficial effects prior to needle penetration. Such effects may be psychological or pharmacological. Factors that influence the pharmacological efficacy of topical anaesthetics include:
• the agent employed
• duration of application
• site of application.

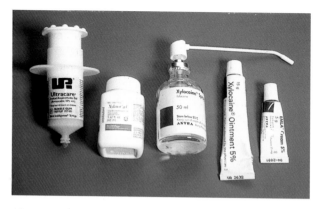

Fig 6-1 Topical anaesthetics are available in a number of formulations.

The agent

Different delivery vehicles are used to administer topical anaesthetics (Fig 6-1). These include:

- aerosols
- ointments
- gels
- lozenges
- tablets
- pastes
- powders
- solutions
- impregnated patches.

Two aspects related to the agent should be considered in relation to efficacy: first the concentration and secondly the anaesthetic agent itself. Different formulations of the same anaesthetic drug need different concentrations to achieve a similar effect. For example, sprays require a higher concentration than patches. The transfer of the anaesthetic through the mucosa is concentration dependent.

A variety of agents are used as topical anaesthetics. The injectable anaesthetics used in the UK are exclusively of the amide group; this class of anaesthetic produces a very low incidence of allergic reactions. Ester local anaesthetics such as benzocaine and amethocaine are used as topical agents. The ester class are more likely to produce allergic reactions than the amides. There is little to choose between most of the different agents as far as efficacy is concerned. Both lidocaine and benzocaine have been shown to exert a pharmacological action when applied topically in the mouth. There is experimental evidence that EMLA cream (see Chapter 3) is more effective than lidocaine alone. This may be due to differences in the effective concentration of the drug. EMLA is not licensed for intraoral use at present.

Duration of application
The depth of penetration of the applied agent is governed by the duration of application. In some studies a 2.5-minute application has been shown to be ineffective yet the same material has achieved an effect at 5 minutes. Thus it may be necessary to maintain the agent in position for 5 minutes in order to achieve a pharmacological effect.

Site
The effectiveness of topical anaesthesia varies in different parts of the mouth. There is evidence that the mandibular buccal fold is more susceptible than the corresponding area in the maxilla. In the maxilla the buccal fold is more readily anaesthetised compared to palatal mucosa after topical application.

Although topical anaesthetics have been shown to reduce the discomfort of infiltration anaesthesia, there is no evidence that they decrease the discomfort of deep regional anaesthetic techniques such as inferior alveolar nerve blocks.

Uses
Normally, topical anaesthesia is used prior to needle penetration for conventional anaesthetic techniques. There are reports of soft tissue surgery procedures performed in the mouth under topical anaesthesia alone. In addition, some reductions in the response of dental pulps to electrical stimulation have been reported following application of topical anaesthesia to the overlying mucosa. Advances in this field should be encouraged. If reliable pulpal anaesthesia could be produced after topical application then needles could be eliminated from the dental local anaesthetic armamentarium. Imagine patient reaction to that!

Jet Injection

Jet injection has been used for many years in dentistry. The technique has been employed as a sole means of anaesthesia and as a method of reducing the

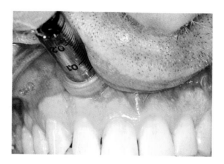

Fig 6-2 A jet injection.

discomfort of subsequent local anaesthetic injection. Jet injection works by forcing anaesthetic through mucosa under pressure (Figs 2-15 and 6-2). A recently described method uses anaesthetic powder. Local anaesthetic solution is employed in most other systems. Some devices accept dental local anaesthetic cartridges; with others the solution has to be drawn up into a reservoir in the injector. The head of the device is placed firmly against mucosa (Fig 6-2) and then the trigger released. This forces the solution through mucosa to produce anaesthesia. The technique has been shown to provide enough anaesthesia in some cases to allow extraction of teeth. On the other hand it is not 100% effective in reducing injection discomfort of needle penetration after surface anaesthesia with jet injection. The efficacy is dependent upon the concentration of local anaesthetic used. Occasionally the patient will experience haematoma formation at the site of use. Another disadvantage is that spillage of anaesthetic solution into the mouth tastes unpleasant.

Intrapapillary Anaesthesia

Intrapapillary injections may be used to obtain localised anaesthesia and haemorrhage control during periodontal surgery. In addition they can be used as a means of obtaining palatal anaesthesia following buccal infiltration. This is particularly useful in children and is described more fully in Chapter 9.

Technique

A short or ultrashort 30-gauge needle should be fitted to the syringe. The needle is inserted at the buccal aspect of the papilla; a site about 2 mm apical to the tip of the papilla is ideal (Fig 6-3). This target should be approached with the needle parallel to the occlusal plane and solution injected slowly;

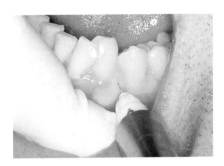

Fig 6-3 An intrapapillary injection.

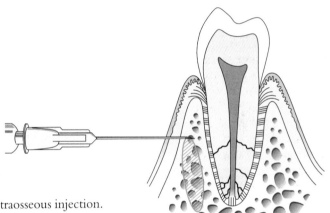

Fig 6-4 The intraosseous injection.

only a small amount of solution (around 0.1 mL) is required. Blanching of the papilla indicates successful deposition.

Intraosseous Anaesthesia

As the name indicates, intraosseous anaesthesia relies upon the deposition of anaesthetic solution directly into the cancellous space (Fig 6-4). Although the technique may be performed with conventional dental local anaesthetic delivery systems, the introduction of specialised equipment has made this method easier to carry out.

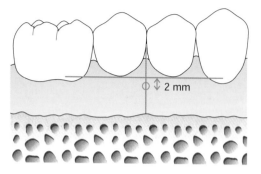

Fig 6-5 The point of penetration for the intraosseous injection is 2 mm below the intersection of the lines illustrated. The horizontal line traverses the gingival margins of the adjacent teeth and the vertical line bisects the interdental papilla.

Technique

The point of penetration is identified (Fig 6-5). It should lie in attached gingiva and is determined by imagining two lines perpendicular to one another. The horizontal line passes along the buccal gingival margins of the teeth. The vertical line bisects the distal interdental papilla of the tooth that is being anaesthetised. The site of perforation is 2 mm apical to the intersection of these lines. If this is located within reflected mucosa an area of attached gingiva coronal to this is chosen. If the approach is made through reflected rather than attached gingiva the bony perforation in the alveolus may be difficult to locate with the needle unless a system with a needle locator is used (see below).

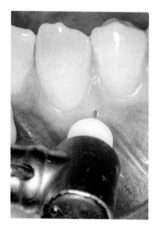

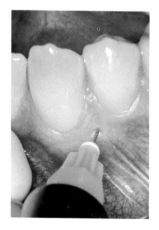

Fig 6-6a The perforator being used during an intraosseous injection.

Fig 6-6b The intraosseous injection being performed.

Deposition of solution through reflected mucosa, although closer to the apex, does not improve the efficacy of intraosseous anaesthesia. Therefore, penetration via attached gingival is recommended. The area of perforation is infiltrated with 0.2 mL of local anaesthetic. The perforator is used one minute later when gingival anaesthesia has occurred. When using the specialised equipment the perforator is advanced through the anaesthetised gingiva and bone using a slowspeed handpiece (Fig 6-6a). A characteristic "give" indicates penetration through to the cancellous bone. Following removal of the perforator, the short (6 mm) 27-gauge needle is inserted through the perforation into the cancellous space (Fig 6-6b). About 1 mL of solution is delivered slowly (over a two-minute period). The technique should be avoided in cases of active periodontal disease, where there is limited attached gingiva or if there is little interradicular bone.

Duration and spread of anaesthesia
The onset of intraosseous anaesthesia is rapid, ranging from 10 to 120 seconds. The success falls off rapidly over an hour and the decline in anaesthesia seems to be more rapid with anterior teeth. The teeth mesial and distal to the tooth of interest will also be anaesthetised in the majority of cases.

Factors governing success
The following factors affect the efficacy of intraosseous anaesthesia
- the choice of anaesthetic solution
- the type of tooth.

1. Anaesthetic solution. The efficacy of intraosseous injections is poor in the absence of a vasoconstrictor. The inclusion of a vasoconstrictor increases both the success and the duration of anaesthesia.
2. Type of tooth. The efficacy of the intraosseous technique varies between teeth. There is greater success with maxillary compared to mandibular molars and this is probably due to differences in the cancellous space between sites.

Advantages of intraosseous anaesthesia
The advantages of intra-osseous anaesthesia over conventional methods include:

- a smaller dose is required
- a smaller area of soft tissue anaesthesia is produced
- the method aids in overcoming failure of conventional techniques.

1. Smaller doses are used than in conventional regional block anaesthesia - around 1 mL is normally sufficient.
2. The amount of soft tissue anaesthesia produced is less than that caused by infiltration and regional block methods and this may reduce the possibility of self-inflicted trauma.
3. When used in combination with inferior alveolar nerve blocks, the method increases the success rate for pulpal anaesthesia compared to the use of the regional block in isolation. Similarly, supplemental anaesthesia via the intra-osseous route may be effective in teeth with irreversible pulpitis where conventional methods have failed.

Disadvantages of intraosseous anaesthesia
The disadvantages of intraosseous anaesthesia include:
- technically more difficult than infiltration anaesthesia
- specialised equipment may be required
- systemic effects may be increased
- post-injection discomfort may be produced
- teeth may be damaged.

1. The method is technically more difficult than infiltration anaesthesia as the entry point made by the perforator must be accurately located. This is simplified with some specialised intraosseous delivery systems that include a locator. This locator remains in position after removal of the perforator and directs the needle into the channel created.
2. Although it is not absolutely essential, specialised equipment makes the method easier.
3. Entry of local anaesthetic and vasoconstrictor into the circulation occurs rapidly following intraosseous anaesthesia and systemic effects attributable to catecholamine-entry into the circulation occur early after injection. Patients may report an increase in heart rate during intraosseous anaesthesia with epinephrine-containing solutions.
4. Post-injection discomfort may occur. Post-operative swelling and an exudate may be produced after intraosseous injections and some patients have perforation sites that are slow to heal.
5. The method may damage teeth. The perforators can penetrate teeth. Fortunately there is a tactile change detectable when dental tissue is encountered and strong pressure has to be used for this to occur.

Intraligamentary (Periodontal Ligament) Anaesthesia

The terms intraligamentary anaesthesia or periodontal ligament anaesthesia

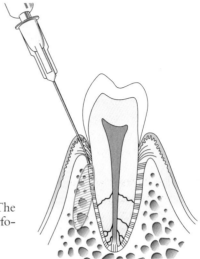

Fig 6-7 The intraligamentary injection. The solution enters the cancellous space via perforations in the socket wall.

are misnomers. Solution injected via the periodontal ligament reaches the pulpal nerve supply by entering the cancellous bone via perforations in the socket wall, not by travelling down the length of the ligament (Fig 6-7). Therefore, this method is a form of intraosseous anaesthesia.

Technique

It is recommended that the site of penetration is swabbed with an antiseptic solution. Efficacy is independent of the syringe and needle gauge used. Although the injection can be performed using either conventional or specialised syringes, it is easier with an intraligamentary syringe. A 30-gauge needle is recommended.

The needle is inserted at the mesiobuccal aspect of the root(s) at 30 degrees to the long axis of the tooth (Fig 6-8). The needle is advanced to maximum

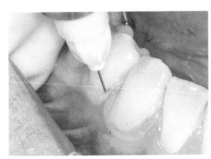

Fig 6-8 An intraligamentary injection.

penetration until it is wedged between the tooth and the alveolar crest. Progression deep into the periodontal ligament is not usually possible. If the bevel of the needle faces the alveolar wall this reduces the chances of blockage. The orientation of the needle, however, is unrelated to the success of the technique. Once the needle is correctly positioned, the solution is injected under backpressure. If resistance to flow of solution is not detected during delivery then efficacy is reduced. It is recommended that 0.2 mL of solution is deposited into the periodontium of each root. When using the specialised syringes the needle should remain in position for about 10 seconds following depression of the lever to allow escape of solution from the cartridge. If the needle is removed too soon then solution spills into the mouth. This tastes unpleasant and may reduce efficacy.

Duration and spread of intraligamentary anaesthesia
The duration of intraligamentary anaesthesia between individuals is marked. The duration of reliable pulpal anaesthesia is around 15 minutes for single-rooted teeth and rather less for molars.

Intraligamentary anaesthesia is not a single-tooth anaesthetic. Spread of anaesthesia to adjacent teeth occurs with both specialised and conventional syringes but appears to happen more frequently with the former type. Spread to adjacent teeth is dependent upon the solution injected, vasoconstrictor-containing solutions affecting more adjacent teeth than plain local anaesthetics.

Factors influencing efficacy
The efficacy of intraligamentary anaesthesia is governed by:
• the choice of solution
• the procedure to be performed on the tooth
• the type of tooth.

1. The anaesthetic solution. Intraligamentary anaesthesia does not occur owing to pulpal ischaemia. It relies on the presence of a local anaesthetic agent. Efficacy is, however, highly dependent upon the presence of a vasoconstrictor. Indeed, success is related more to the concentration of the vasoconstrictor employed than to the anaesthetic agent used.
2. The operative procedure. Like most anaesthetic techniques, intraligamentary anaesthesia is most effective prior to dental extractions and least effective for endodontic procedures.
3. The type of tooth. The efficacy of intraligamentary anaesthesia varies between the teeth. Efficacy is greater for those teeth with both mesial and

distal contact points. Canines can be resistant. This is probably owing to the distance the solution must travel from alveolar crest to canine apex. The teeth for which it is most difficult to achieve pulpal anaesthesia are lower incisors. This is partly owing to the paucity of perforations in the alveolus in this region. In addition, there is little cancellous bone in the interdental space in the lower incisor area.

Advantages of intraligamentary anaesthesia
The advantages of intraligamentary anaesthesia compared with conventional methods include:
- smaller dose required
- rapid onset of anaesthesia
- the method aids in overcoming failure of conventional techniques
- only a small area of soft tissue is anaesthetised
- it is useful in the mandible for patients with bleeding diatheses.

1. Smaller doses are required compared to conventional infiltration and block anaesthesia. The normal dose is 0.2 mL per root.
2. The onset of anaesthesia is rapid. Anaesthesia is achieved within thirty seconds and can be immediate.
3. The method overcomes failed conventional anaesthesia. Intraligamentary injections have been shown to be successful in overcoming failed inferior alveolar nerve blocks.
4. There is limited soft tissue anaesthesia. The elimination of unwanted soft tissue anaesthesia can be beneficial particularly in the mandible. This may make four-quadrant dentistry more acceptable. In addition, it is useful in overcoming the problems of self-inflicted trauma that may occur in anaesthetised regions in children. It should be pointed out that some soft tissue anaesthesia does occur with this method and warnings concerning the dangers of self-inflicted trauma should still be given.
5. The technique can be used for mandibular anaesthesia in patients with bleeding diatheses. Regional block injections are hazardous in patients with bleeding diatheses and may require administration of pre-operative supplements such as Factor VIII. Intraligamentary anaesthesia injections may be given safely without such prophylaxis.

Disadvantages of intraligamentary anaesthesia
The disadvantages of intraligamentary anaesthesia include:
- the production of a bacteraemia
- increased systemic effects
- peri- and postinjection discomfort can occur

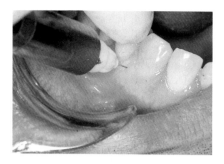

Fig 6-9 The intraligamentary injection can be given via the interdental papilla. This reduces the bacteraemia produced by this type of injection when compared to the approach via the gingival sulcus.

- damage to dental and periodontal tissues can be caused
- damage to equipment may be produced.

1. Injecting via the periodontal ligament produces a significant bacteraemia. Thus, intraligamentary anaesthesia represents a potential cause of endocarditis in "at-risk" groups. The bacteraemia may be reduced by modifying the injection technique. This alteration involves approaching the crest of the alveolus through the gingival tissue (Fig 6-9) rather than via the gingival crevice.

2. The entry of local anaesthetic and vasoconstrictor into circulation is rapid following intraligamentary anaesthesia. Direct entry of the needle into the lumen of a blood vessel is unlikely using the periodontal ligament technique. The solution reaches the vasculature quickly, however, via the socket walls. Entry into the circulation has been shown to be as rapid as intravenous administration after intraligamentary anaesthesia. This rapid entry can increase unwanted systemic effects.

3. Peri- and postinjection discomfort can occur. The discomfort of intraligamentary injection varies markedly between individuals; some patients find the method more painful than conventional infiltration anaesthesia. The method may produce postoperative discomfort. This may be due to tooth extrusion, which causes a traumatic occlusion.

4. Intraligamentary anaesthesia may damage dental and periodontal tissues. Animal studies have shown dramatic reductions in pulpal blood flow after intraligamentary injections. This has not been demonstrated conclusively in humans. Similarly, animal studies have suggested that intraligamentary anaesthesia can produce damage to unerupted teeth in the zone of injection. Certainly, local anaesthetics are toxic to enamel organs. Nevertheless, no such developmental problems have been reported in humans. Intraligamentary injections do produce changes in the periodontal tissues. This is partly due to physical injury by the needle. Reversible dam-

age occurs to the ligament, cementum and alveolar bone. Animal studies suggest that normal anatomy returns within two weeks. One area where irreversible change may occur is the interdental septal crest when intraligamentary injections are administered on either side of this bone - that is the distal aspect of one tooth and the mesial aspect of the adjacent distal tooth. Crestal bone may become necrotic under such a circumstance. Thus intraligamentary injections should be avoided on both sides of the same interdental septum when adjacent teeth are undergoing restorative dentistry.

5. Injection equipment may be damaged. The forces generated during intraligamentary injections are such that glass local anaesthetic cartridges may be broken. Suitable protection, such as a plastic sheath, should be used around the cartridge to prevent damage to patient and operator. Plastic cartridges should not be used, as the pressures involved will cause distortion leading to escape of anaesthetic solution from the plunger rather than the needle.

Intraseptal Anaesthesia

Intraseptal anaesthesia is, in a sense, a hybrid of intraligamentary and intraosseous anaesthesia. It achieves an effect identical to intraligamentary injection, but the technique is different. A short 27-gauge needle is inserted

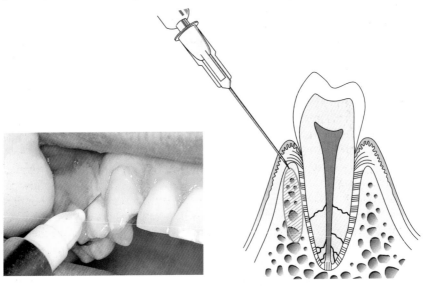

Fig 6-10 An intraseptal injection.   **Fig 6-11** The intraseptal injection.

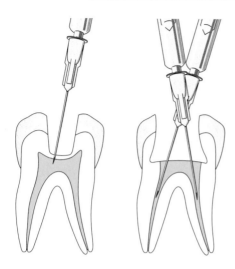

Fig 6-12 Intrapulpal anaesthesia relies upon a tight fit of the needle. This may be via a small perforation in the pulp chamber or if a large defect exists in a multi-rooted tooth the needle must be inserted to maximum penetration along each root.

into the buccal interdental papilla, injecting while it is directed toward the bone (Figs 6-10 and 6-11). Once bone is contacted the needle is advanced into the bone and 0.2 mL of solution injected. The technique may be used instead of the intraligamentary method if the periodontal condition is poor.

Intrapulpal Anaesthesia

Technique
This method of anaesthesia relies on deposition of solution directly into the pulp canals. Usually it will be administered following the injection of an anaesthetic solution by another route. It is essential that the solution is injected into the pulp under pressure. If a defect is not present, an opening into the pulp should be made with a small round bur. This access point should allow the snug fit of the needle. If a large opening is present in the pulp chamber then the needle must be advanced into the canal until the fit is tight (Fig 6-12). The important point is that the injection must be administered under pressure. Around 0.2 mL of solution is injected. A number of methods of obliterating a large pulpal opening may be tried, such as using gutta-percha or a cotton pledget. The only way to ensure no back flow is to introduce the needle through a small pulpal opening.

Spread of intrapulpal anaesthesia
Material injected into a pulp canal rarely reaches adjacent pulp canals. Therefore, in multirooted teeth, separate injections at each canal are needed. In

addition, other factors determine that each root canal must receive independent injections (see below).

Factors influencing efficacy

It appears that the efficacy of intrapulpal anaesthesia is independent of the solution used. There is ample evidence that saline is as effective as a local anaesthetic solution, indicating that the method achieves its effect by pulpal ischaemia. This adds further importance to the fact that each canal must be injected independently.

Advantages of intrapulpal anaesthesia

The advantages of intrapulpal anaesthesia are:
- success is independent of the solution
- the method aids in overcoming failed conventional methods
- single tooth anaesthesia may be obtained
- there are minimal systemic effects.

1. As mentioned above, the method does not require a local anaesthetic.
2. The method provides a useful means of overcoming failure in teeth where conventional techniques have been unsuccessful.
3. Intrapulpal anaesthesia uniquely could provide single-tooth anaesthesia. As it is normally administered after failure of another method this possibility is excluded in most cases.
4. The systemic effects of intrapulpal anaesthesia appear to be negligible. Epinephrine-containing solutions when injected via the pulp produce minimal changes in comparison with similar doses injected via the periodontal ligament. In addition, as the technique is independent of the solution, the use of an appropriate material will further reduce systemic effects.

Disadvantages of intrapulpal anaesthesia

The disadvantages of intrapulpal anaesthesia include:
- discomfort may be produced
- application of the method is limited.

1. Intrapulpal injections can be painful.
2. The technique has limited indications as it involves pulpal exposure. Thus it is useful only for oral surgery and endodontic procedures.

Transcutaneous Electronic Nerve Stimulation

Non-pharmacological methods of anaesthesia, such as transcutaneous elec-

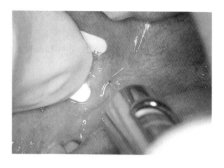

Fig 6-13 Transcutaneous electronic nerve stimulation being used to reduce the discomfort of an inferior alveolar nerve block injection. The electrodes are attached to the operator's gloved thumb and the patient controls the frequency and amplitude of the stimulus.

tronic nerve stimulation (TENS), have been used both as a means of reducing the discomfort of injections (Fig 6-13) and as a method of achieving pulpal anaesthesia.

The technique involves the use of electrical leads applied either to the region of injection or close to the nerve supplying the tooth in question. This application can be either intra- or extraoral and the leads may be attached to the operator's finger or the patient's mucosa or skin. The frequency and amplitude of the stimulation from the electrodes is controlled by a console. The frequency is normally preset but the patient controls the amplitude. The patient adjusts the strength of the signal until a pleasant vibratory sensation is experienced. As accommodation occurs, the patient gradually increases the amplitude of the current. TENS has been shown to decrease the discomfort of infiltration and inferior alveolar nerve block injections. This method of anaesthesia can provide pain control for operative dentistry in some patients. However, success is poor for endodontic procedures.

Conclusions

- A number of supplementary techniques other than infiltration and regional block anaesthesia can be used in both jaws.
- Some techniques, such as topical anaesthesia, are used to reduce injection discomfort.
- Some techniques, such as intraosseous and intraligamentary injections, are used to overcome failed conventional methods of dental anaesthesia.

Further Reading

Nusstein J, Reader A, Nist R, Beck M, Meyers WJ. Anesthetic efficacy of the supplemental intraosseous injection of 2% lidocaine with 1:100,000 epinephrine in irreversible pulpitis. J Endodontics 1998;24:487-491.

Smith GN, Walton RE, Abbott BJ. Clinical evaluation of periodontal ligament anesthesia using a pressure syringe. J Amer Dent Assoc 1983;107:953-956.

VanGheluwe J, Walton R. Intrapulpal injection. Factors related to effectiveness. Oral Surg Oral Med Oral Path 1997;83:38-40.

Chapter 7
Safety

Aim

The aim of this chapter is to discuss factors related to the safety of local anaesthesia in dentistry.

Outcome

After reading this chapter you should have an understanding of important medical conditions and drug interactions which impact upon the use of local anaesthesia. In addition, you will have an awareness of the safe maximum doses.

Introduction and Terminology

Local anaesthetics have a remarkable safety record in dentistry. This should not lead to complacency in their use. Some groups of the population are more at risk of unwanted effects than others. Among these individuals with increased risk are children, the elderly and medically compromised patients. The cessation of general anaesthetic services in dental practice means that more treatments are being provided for children under local anaesthesia in dentistry. Therefore, safety issues are of increasing importance. As with all adverse reactions, prevention is better than cure.

A major factor in reducing adverse reactions is eliciting a thorough medical and drug history from the patient before injection. The importance of history taking cannot be overemphasised.

The unwanted effects of dental local anaesthesia can occur due to:
- physical trauma
- chemical trauma
- inappropriate site of deposition
- toxicity
- allergy
- an underlying medical condition
- drug interactions.

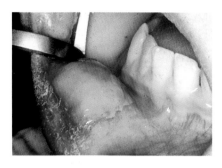

Fig 7-1 A self-inflicted injury following an inferior alveolar nerve block.

Physical Trauma

Trauma can occur at two stages. First, the needle may cause it. Secondly, it may arise as a result of self-injury in an anaesthetised area.

During regional block techniques the needle may damage the nerve trunk. This can cause long-lasting altered sensation, either anaesthesia or paraesthesia. The management of this problem is discussed in Chapter 8. Penetration of a blood vessel may produce bleeding into muscle (for example, the medial pterygoid may be traumatised during an inferior alveolar nerve block). This may produce muscle spasm resulting in trismus.

Self-inflicted trauma may occur if the patient inadvertently, or deliberately, bites an anaesthetised area. This can be a potential problem with children and therefore the patient and parent should be advised about the dangers of biting the area anaesthetised (Fig 7-1).

Chemical Trauma

In high concentration local anaesthetics may damage nerves. This can result in long-lasting altered sensation and is discussed in Chapter 8.

Inappropriate Site of Deposition

Occasionally, local anaesthetics are injected in the wrong place such as intravascularly or into the parotid gland.

Intravascular injection
The incidence of intravascular injection varies from site to site in the mouth. The routine use of an aspirating technique is recommended to reduce the

chances of inadvertent injection into a blood vessel. During inferior alveolar nerve block injections, incidences of positive aspirates up to 20% of injections have been reported. In other sites, such as the maxillary buccal sulcus, the figure is around 2%. Intravascular injection may cause:

• pain
• localised blanching
• cranial effects
• systemic effects.

Although the needle may penetrate arteries or veins, it is unusual to enter the lumen of an artery. This is because arteries tend to slip away from the needle unless firmly attached to bone. Entry of a local anaesthetic into an artery will cause localised pain and blanching. Transport of the local anaesthetic in a cranial direction has occasionally caused transient blindness in one eye, limitation in eye movement leading to double vision, and temporary deafness. The most dramatic effect is transfer of material into the brain causing transient hemiplegia. Fortunately, although reported, this is an extremely rare occurrence. Nevertheless, it does dramatically illustrate the importance of aspiration prior to and during injection.

Inadvertent injection into a vein is more common than intra-arterial deposition. Systemic distribution of the anaesthetic agent and any added vasoconstrictor would follow intravenous injection. This may produce toxicity and this is described below.

Injection into parotid gland
The facial nerve traverses the parotid gland. Accidental injection deep to the parotid sheath during an inferior alveolar nerve block will introduce solution into the substance of the gland. This can result in anaesthetic solution affecting the facial nerve. Motor nerves are susceptible to the actions of local anaesthetics. If the facial nerve is affected, the patient will experience hemifacial paresis. The major problem that results is inability of the patient to close the eyelids on the affected side. This is not a dangerous condition so long as the affected eye is protected during the duration of the paralysis. The paralysis will resolve as the effect of the anaesthetic wears off. Clearly, this scenario is best avoided and steps can be taken to minimise the chances of hemifacial paralysis occurring. Ensuring that the needle has contacted bone prior to administration of an inferior-alveolar nerve block should reduce the chances of entering the parotid gland. The rapid deposition of large quantities of local anaesthetic solution in the maxillary buccal sulcus may also cause temporary problems in eyelid closure. In this case the entire facial nerve has

not been affected and the paralysis is more localised. Once again, the eye must be protected until motor function is restored.

Toxicity

Toxicity may be due to either the local anaesthetic or to any contained vasoconstrictor. The dose combinations found in dental local anaesthetic solutions are such that it is easier to achieve toxic levels of the anaesthetic compared with the vasoconstrictor. Idiosyncratic reactions may occur in some individuals, however, leading to toxic effects of the vasoconstrictor. If a toxic reaction occurs it is important to determine the causative agent, as the treatment differs (Table 7-1). When the effect is due to the local anaesthetic, the patient is laid flat to combat circulatory collapse. When epinephrine toxicity occurs, the patient is sat upright to reduce cerebral blood pressure. Toxicity to local anaesthesia can be the result of the following:
• an intravascular injection
• overdosage
• the patient's inability to metabolise.

Prevention of toxicity is better than cure. Preventive measures include:
• aspiration before and during injection
• calculation of safe maximum dose before treatment begins
• slow injection.

Table 7-1. **Treatment of toxicity.**

Local anaesthetic toxicity	Epinephrine toxicity
stop treatment	stop treatment
lie patient flat	place patient supine or erect
administer oxygen	administer oxygen if not hyperventilating
give intravenous fluids	reassure patient
give intravenous anticonvulsants	
basic life support	

Intravascular injection

It was mentioned above that intravenous injection could lead to systemic distribution of relatively high doses of both anaesthetic and vasoconstrictor. As all excitable tissues are susceptible to the action of local anaesthetics then unwanted effects may occur. As far as the anaesthetic agent is concerned the most susceptible organs are the brain and the heart.

Local anaesthetic toxicity of the central nervous system begins as excitation as the first effect is on inhibitory fibre activity. This presents as restlessness and tremors. Later stages of toxicity produce central nervous system depression that can lead to unconsciousness and ultimately the fatal condition of respiratory arrest (Fig 7-2).

There is sufficient local anaesthetic contained in a cartridge to produce toxic levels of the agent in the central nervous system in children and small adults. This is illustrated in Fig 7-3.

The commonly used local anaesthetics affect the heart. At low doses cardiac output may be increased owing to a disinhibition of autonomic nerve activity. At toxic doses there is a direct depressant effect resulting in circulatory collapse.

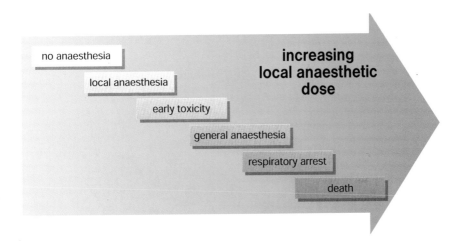

Fig 7-2 What happens when the dose of local anaesthetic increases.

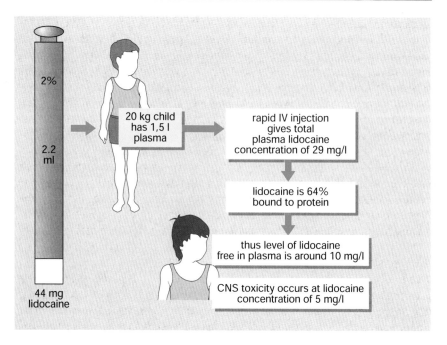

Fig 7-3 An illustration of how easy it is to overdose if a direct intravascular injection is administered in a child.

Table 7-2. **Signs of epinephrine overdose.**

fear
anxiety
restlessness
headache
trembling
sweating
weakness
dizziness
pallor
respiratory difficulties
palpitations

Epinephrine toxicity will induce effects similar to those experienced in fright (Table 7-2). In addition, vasoconstrictors may produce adverse effects on the cardiovascular system. Epinephrine increases cardiac output by increasing both the rate and force of contraction of the heart owing to $beta_1$-adrenergic stimulation. This may lead to an increase in systolic blood pressure. Alpha-adrenergic stimulation causes vasoconstriction of peripheral vessels that is useful in providing haemostasis. $Beta_2$-adrenergic stimulation causes a vasodilatation in blood vessels in other organs such as the liver and skeletal muscle. This latter effect can reduce diastolic blood pressure. In addition to direct effects on the heart and blood vessels, epinephrine produces metabolic changes that can affect cardiovascular function. One metabolic effect that can influence cardiovascular function is the effect of epinephrine on plasma potassium levels. Epinephrine reduces plasma potassium and large shifts in the concentration of this ion can lead to dysrhythmias.

Overdose
Ultimately, all of a local anaesthetic dose will enter the blood stream to allow metabolism and excretion. One factor governing the plasma level is the total dose administered. Normally in dental practice the maximum safe dose of a local anaesthetic is not injected. In certain circumstances, however, volumes approaching the maximum recommended may be used. This may be a particular problem with children or small adults as the dose administered

Table 7-3. **Relationship of one-tenth of a cartridge to the maximum recommended dose of local anaesthetic agents.**

Drug	Cartridge volume	Maximum dose	Amount in one-tenth of a cartridge
2% lidocaine	1.8 mL	4.4 mg/kg	3.6 mg
2% lidocaine	2.0 mL	4.4 mg/kg	4.0 mg
2% lidocaine	2.2 mL	4.4 mg/kg	4.4 mg
2% mepivacaine	2.0 mL	4.4 mg/kg	4.0 mg
3% mepivacaine	2.0 mL	4.4 mg/kg	6.0 mg
3% prilocaine	2.2 mL	6.0 mg/kg	6.6 mg
4% prilocaine	2.2 mL	6.0 mg/kg	8.8 mg
4% articaine	1.7 mL	7.0 mg/kg	6.8 mg
4% articaine	2.0 mL	7.0 mg/kg	8.0 mg

is governed by the weight of the patient. In addition, the elderly may be more likely to suffer toxic reactions owing to metabolic factors explained below. The maximum recommended dose for all of the commonly used local anaesthetics is given in Table 7-3. As a working rule, a maximum of a tenth of a cartridge per kilogram is recommended for healthy patients. This suggestion is not sacrosanct but is a useful practical guide. This approach simplifies the calculation when combinations of different solutions are used in the same patient. It is important to remember that different local anaesthetics will have an additive effect in relation to toxicity. In other words, when the maximum dose of one agent has been reached that is the most of any local anaesthetic that may be used. Switching to another agent does not mean that further cartridges can be employed.

It might be thought that the addition of a vasoconstrictor to a local anaesthetic means that a greater dose of the local anaesthetic could be administered, as the vasoconstrictor inhibits entry of the anaesthetic into the blood stream. Although a vasoconstrictor may delay the entry of the anaesthetic it has little effect on the peak plasma concentration. Epinephrine alters the distribution of blood in the body and sends relatively more to the brain (a site vulnerable to local anaesthetic toxicity). This means that the addition of epinephrine has the potential to increase central nervous system toxicity. Thus the maximum safe doses mentioned above should be used whether or not a vasoconstrictor is present.

Metabolic disorders

As mentioned above, local anaesthetics are absorbed from their site of deposition, metabolised and excreted. Most of the amide agents administered by injection in dental local anaesthesia are metabolised in the liver. Prilocaine also undergoes some metabolism in the lung. The main exception is articaine, which undergoes initial metabolism in the plasma by esterases.

As the liver is the main organ involved in local anaesthetic metabolism, any condition that affects hepatic activity will influence the metabolism of local anaesthetics. When there is no metabolic activity at all, in other words in a patient with no hepatic function, then all the injected dose will appear in the circulation. As illustrated in Fig 7-3, there is enough anaesthetic in a cartridge to produce central nervous system toxicity in some patients if it is not metabolised. It is unlikely that a patient with no hepatic activity will be encountered in dental practice. If a patient has a degree of hepatic impairment this must be considered when assessing the maximum dose allowed. Indeed, where liver function is severely compromised discussion with the supervising physician is essential.

Disease and drugs (such as alcohol) are not the only factors that can reduce the performance of the liver. Age affects hepatic function. As a working rule, metabolic activity of the liver in a patient aged 65 years is approximately half of that in a 25-year-old. This should be taken into account when estimating maximum doses.

Methaemoglobinaemia

Methaemoglobinaemia is a toxic effect that may be produced by some local anaesthetics, principally prilocaine. This is the conversion of haemoglobin to methaemoglobin owing to the presence of iron in the ferric rather than the ferrous form. It may produce cyanosis but is unlikely to occur at normal clinical doses in adults, although small doses may produce this phenomenon in children. The condition is treated by the intravenous injection of methylene blue.

Allergy

An allergic reaction to the amide group of local anaesthetics is extremely rare. Members of the ester group are more likely to produce allergy. In the past, the preservatives used in local anaesthetics could produce an allergic response but most modern solutions are preservative-free. The reducing agent in epinephrine-containing solutions may produce unwanted effects in those with sulphur allergies. Although the incidence of allergy is rare, it does occur in some individuals and a history of a rash or difficulty in breathing following the administration of a dental local anaesthetic should be taken seriously. Patients reporting such symptoms should be referred for specialist investigation to a dermatologist or clinical immunologist. Such tests will provide two important pieces of information. First, evidence will be provided relating to which local anaesthetic, if any, to avoid. Secondly, it will inform the dentist which solutions can be used safely in the patient. Fortunately, most reports of allergy prove to be episodes of fainting or stress reactions.

In addition to allergic reactions to the constituents of the solution, there is another potential allergen that may be encountered in dental local anaesthesia. This is latex. As mentioned in Chapter 2, the plungers in some local anaesthetic cartridges contain latex. The use of such cartridges has produced life-threatening anaphylactic shock in patients with severe latex allergy. Fortunately, there are latex-free cartridges available.

Table 7-4. **Recommended ACTion with medical conditions.**

Medical condition	Local anaesthetic drug	Epinephrine	Felypressin	Intra-ligamentary-Injections	Deep block Injections	TENS
Unstable angina		A	C			
Severe dysrhythmia		A	C			
Endocarditis risk- no prophylaxis				A		
Demand pace-maker						A
Other cardiac disease		C	C			
Allergy to local anaesthetic	A					
Liver disease	C					
Malignant hyperthermia	T					
Phaechromo-cytoma		A				
Pregnancy	C		T			
Epilepsy						A
Bleeding diathesis- no prophylaxis					A	

Key
A = **A**void: severe reactions may occur
C = **C**aution: an adverse interaction can occur in dental practice (see text for specific conditions and drugs involved)
T = **T**heoretical interaction unlikely in dental practice at normal clinical doses

Medically Compromised Patients

There are two aspects concerning medical conditions that should be considered in relation to local anaesthesia. These are:
• the underlying condition
• drug interactions.

The dentist needs to know how to **act** in such cases. Indeed, the word ACT is a useful acronym in this regard.

> A = avoid use
> C = caution to be used
> T = theoretical interaction.

The suggested ACTions are summarised in Table 7.4 and the conditions and drug interactions are discussed below.

Underlying medical conditions

Metabolic concerns arising from liver disease that might lead to toxicity were mentioned above. Cardiac disease impacts upon the use of vasoconstrictors, especially epinephrine. Heart problems that are of concern are uncontrolled arrhythmias and unstable angina. Avoidance of epinephrine is wise in such cases and the use of another vasoconstrictor such as felypressin is recom-

Table 7-5. **Recommended ACTion with concurrent drug therapy.**

Drug	"Social" /abuse drugs	Benzodia- zepines	Antimicro- bials	Anticonvul- sants	Cardio- vascular drugs	CNS drugs
Local anaesthetic drug		C	C	T	C	
Vasoconstrictors	C				C	C

Key
A = **A**void: severe reactions may occur
C = **C**aution: an adverse interaction can occur in dental practice (see text for specific conditions and drugs involved)
T = **T**heoretical interaction unlikely in dental practice at normal clinical doses

mended. Even the use of felypressin is not without hazard in patients with cardiac disease. At high doses this drug produces coronary artery vasoconstriction. Thus, a maximum of three cartridges of a felypressin-containing solution is suggested for adults with cardiac disease.

When treating patients with other cardiac conditions, avoidance of epinephrine is not essential. However, sensible dose reductions should be employed. No more than two cartridges of an epinephrine-containing solution in adults are recommended in these cases.

There is a suspicion that lidocaine may produce malignant hyperthermia in susceptible individuals, but this appears to be unlikely. The rare condition of phaeochromocytoma, which is a catecholamine-producing tumour of the adrenal glands, is unlikely to be encountered in dental practice. This condition is a contraindication to the use of epinephrine.

Felypressin has an oxytocic effect on the uterus. That means it can produce uterine contraction. The dose needed to induce labour is equivalent to around 100 dental cartridges of a 0.03IU/mL solution. Therefore, this particular effect is not a concern in dental practice. Local anaesthetics will cross the placenta. The drugs used in dentistry differ in the amount of diffusion across this organ. Prilocaine diffuses the most and therefore is not the best choice in the pregnant female. Bupivacaine has the potential to produce the most foetal hypoxia and thus is not the ideal local anaesthetic to administer during pregnancy.

Other medical conditions that interfere with different aspects of local anaesthesia include the presence of demand-type pacemakers and epilepsy. Both of these are contraindications to the use of electronic dental anaesthesia such as TENS.

The use of deep regional block injections should be avoided in patients with bleeding diatheses such as haemophilia unless appropriate prophylaxis (Factor VIII) has been provided. The use intraligamentary anaesthesia is safe in these patients. This latter technique should not be used in patients at risk of endocarditis in the absence of prophylactic antibiotics, as intraligamentary injections produce a significant bacteraemia.

Drug interactions
Drug interactions may occur with either local anaesthetics or vasoconstrictors. Indeed the relationship of the local anaesthetic and the vasoconstrictor

is an example of a useful interaction as the latter drug increases the effectiveness of the former.

Local anaesthetics
Drugs that might interact with local anaesthetic agents used in dentistry include:
anticonvulsants
antimicrobials
benzodiazepines
beta-adrenergic blockers
calcium-channel blockers.

Anticonvulsants
Lidocaine and phenytoin both depress cardiac activity. This is probably only important at high doses.

Antimicrobials
Drugs such as sulfonamide antibacterials can exacerbate the methaemoglobinaemia produced by prilocaine. This may even occur following topical application of the local anaesthetic.

Protease inhibitor drugs used in the management of HIV raise the plasma levels of lidocaine and potentially increase cardiotoxicity.

Benzodiazepines
An advantageous drug interaction is that between midazolam and lidocaine. The benzodiazepine reduces the central nervous system toxicity of the local anaesthetic. It should be mentioned that this benefit does not apply to all benzodiazepine/local anaesthetic combinations. For example, diazepam raises the serum levels of bupivacaine, thus increasing the toxicity of the local anaesthetic.

Beta-adrenergic blockers
Beta-adrenergic-blocking drugs increase the toxicity of amide local anaesthetics by decreasing hepatic blood flow and inhibiting liver enzymes. This is not an absolute contraindication to the use of local anaesthetics. The maximum dose administered, however, should be reduced in patients taking beta-blockers. No more than two cartridges of an epinephrine-containing solution in adults is recommended (see below).

103

Calcium-channel blockers

Verapamil increases the toxicity of lidocaine. Again, this is not an absolute contraindication to use. However, dose limitation should be exercised. Similarly, calcium-channel blockers increase the cardiotoxicity of the long-acting local anaesthetic bupivacaine.

Vasoconstrictors

Drugs that interfere with epinephrine include:
- beta-adrenergic blockers
- diuretics
- calcium-channel blockers
- drugs acting on the central nervous system
  - anti-Parkinson drugs
  - antidepressant drugs
  - general anaesthetics
  - drugs of abuse.

Beta-adrenergic blockers

As mentioned above, beta-adrenergic stimulation leads to a fall in diastolic blood pressure and alpha-adrenergic effects cause a rise in systolic blood pressure. When the beta-effects are blocked, alpha-adrenergic stimulation may lead to an unopposed increase in systolic blood pressure, which could cause a cerebro-vascular accident such as a stroke. Thus, excessive levels of epinephrine should be avoided in patients taking beta-adrenergic blockers. Beta-adrenoceptor blockers protect the heart from the increase in rate caused by beta-adrenergic stimulation produced by exogenous epinephrine.

Diuretics

Diuretic drugs may interfere with some of the metabolic actions of epinephrine. For example, the catecholamine decreases the levels of plasma potassium. Non-potassium sparing diuretics can increase epinephrine-induced hypokalaemia. This is not an absolute contraindication to the use of epinephrine. However, it is probably wise to limit the dose to one or two cartridges in adults taking these diuretics.

Calcium-channel blockers

As is the case with diuretics, calcium-channel blocking drugs may increase epinephrine-induced hypokalaemia and limitation to one or two cartridges in adults receiving this type of medication is wise.

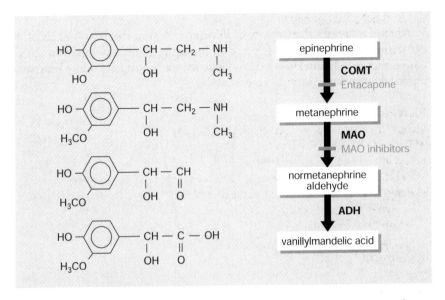

Fig 7-4 The metabolism of epinephrine showing the points of interaction of some anti-Parkinson and antidepressant drugs.

Anti-Parkinson drugs

The metabolism of epinephrine is shown in Fig 7-4. In addition, the sites of action of drugs that interfere with this metabolic process are demonstrated in Fig 7-4. As the anti-Parkinson drug entacapone affects the action of catechol-O-methyl transferase (COMT, the enzyme which initiates exogenous epinephrine metabolism), this drug could be problematic. Although there are no data as yet concerning the influence of entacapone on the adverse effects of epinephrine in dental local anaesthetics, it is wise to be cautious with epinephrine-containing local anaesthetics in patients taking this drug; one cartridge may be a wise limit in adults.

Antidepressant drugs

It is apparent from Fig 7-4 that monoamine oxidase inhibitors exert their effect at a late stage in epinephrine metabolism (after COMT) and therefore combined use is not a concern.

Tricyclic antidepressants decrease the re-uptake of epinephrine into nerve cells. This can increase the pressor effects of the catecholamine. This is only a concern at high doses of epinephrine and does not appear to affect the administration of one or two cartridges of local anaesthetics in adult patients.

General anaesthetics
Volatile general anaesthetic agents such as halothane increase the cardiac sensitivity to catecholamines and a reduction of 50% in the maximum dose of epinephrine injected during dental local anaesthesia is advised.

Drugs of abuse
Drugs which posses sympathomimetic properties will increase epinephrine toxicity. Examples of such drugs include the illicit substances amphetamines, cannabis and cocaine. It is wise to limit the amount of, or avoid, epinephrine-containing local anaesthetics in individuals who have abused these substances within the previous 24 hours.

Staff Safety

It is not only the patient who is at risk from local anaesthesia. The dentist and staff are in danger of needlestick injury. Once a needle has been used on a patient it has the potential to be a lethal weapon if it stabs another individual. Excellent cross-infection and needlestick prevention protocols are essential in every surgery to prevent transmission of blood-borne diseases such as hepatitis and HIV. A used needle should never be resheathed by hand. When non-disposable syringe systems are used it is best to remove the needle using instrumentation as shown in Fig 7-5. As mentioned in Chapter 2, some designs of syringe eliminate the need for needle detachment at the end of injection (Figs 7-6a-c). Use of this type of syringe has been shown to reduce the incidence of needle-stick injury.

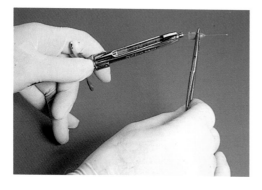

Fig 7-5 Needles should not be removed by the fingers after use. An instrument may be employed as shown here if a non-disposable syringe system is being used.

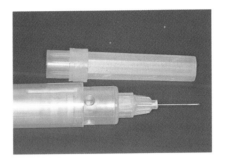
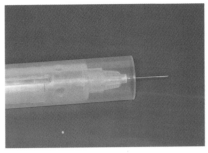
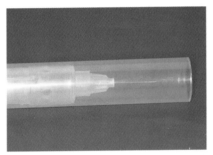

Fig 7-6a-c The use of disposable systems with inbuilt needle protective sheaths reduces the incidence of needlestick injuries.

Conclusions

- Serious side effects of local anaesthesia are rare.
- The potential for toxic reactions exists in children and the elderly.
- It is essential to take a full drug and medical history before injection.

Further Reading

Perusse R, Goulet J-P, Turcotte J-Y. Contraindications to the use of vasoconstrictors in dentistry. Pt 1. Oral Surg Oral Med Oral Path 1992;74:679-686.

Roberts GJ, Simmons NA, Longhurst P, Hewitt PB. Bacteraemia following local anaesthetic injections in children. Br Dent J 1998;185:295-298.

Zakrzewska JM, Greenwood I, Jackson J. Introducing safety syringes into a UK dental school: A controlled study. Br Dent J 2001;190:88-92.

Chapter 8
Trouble-shooting

Aim

The aim of this chapter is to describe methods of overcoming failed local anaesthesia and of dealing with pre- and post-anaesthetic problems.

Outcome

After reading this chapter you should have an understanding of the reasons for anaesthetic failure. You should have developed approaches to overcoming failure and to reducing the problems caused by local anaesthetic administration.

Introduction

This chapter will consider the reasons why local anaesthetics fail. An approach to the failed local anaesthetic will be described. In addition, problems independent of underlying medical conditions that may be encountered before and after injection will be discussed. The medical problems of importance in relation to local anaesthesia are described in Chapter 7.

Pre-anaesthetic Problems

Problems may arise before the provision of anaesthesia owing to:
• patient anxiety
• inability to deliver the solution at the appropriate site.

Patient anxiety
Patient anxiety may lead to the following problems:
• fainting
• reduced anaesthetic efficacy.

1. Fainting
Fainting may occur before, during or after local anaesthetic administration. The patient develops pallor, may sweat and complain of nausea. They may

experience tingling in the extremities and ultimately lose consciousness. The pulse may be rapid in the early stages but then it becomes slow and weak. The cause is a reduction in cranial blood supply. The remedy is to place the patient supine. Recovery is rapid after this manœuvre. If consciousness is not regained quickly then another cause of unconsciousness due to a medical problem must be suspected and appropriate treatment given.

The chances of fainting can be reduced by dealing with the patient in a confident, calm and reassuring manner. In addition, injections should not be administered with the subject in an upright position. Tilting the dental chair backwards or having it flat will maintain the blood supply to the brain.

2. Reduced anaesthetic efficacy
Local anaesthesia is more successful in the relaxed patient. Relaxation can be produced by pharmacological or non-pharmacological methods. The use of conscious sedation to reduce anxiety is discussed below in relation to failure of anaesthesia.

Inability to deliver the solution at the appropriate site
Some techniques require the patient to open widely in order to gain access to the injection site. Examples are the standard approach to the inferior alveolar nerve and palatal injections. If the patient cannot open the mouth widely then this may be problematic. Failure to open the mouth may be due to trismus as a result of pathology or may be stress-related. If the trismus is due to infection of the floor of the mouth and there is dysphagea the patient should be referred for specialist management. Such patients should not be treated in general dental practice as this scenario can rapidly lead on to severe embarrassment of the airway.

Other causes of trismus can be overcome by choosing alternative local anaesthetic techniques. The palatal tissues may be approached via the buccal papillae as described in Chapter 9. Similarly, the inferior alveolar nerve can be anaesthetised in the patient with trismus using the Akinosi closed-mouth method described in Chapter 5. This latter method also overcomes problems due to a large or uncontrollable tongue impinging on the area of needle penetration used during the standard inferior alveolar nerve block. Failure to open the mouth owing to anxiety may be overcome using conscious sedation.

Failure of Local Anaesthesia

Local anaesthesia is not 100% successful in dentistry. The reasons for failure of a local anaesthetic can be classified as:
- anatomical
- pathological
- pharmaceutical
- pharmacological
- psychological
- technical.

These causes are discussed below. Fortunately, in many cases, failure is corrected simply by repeating the initial injection. Thus the first stage in dealing with a failed administration is to repeat it.

Anatomical Causes of Failure

Anatomical causes of failure may be owing to:
- bony barriers to diffusion
- variations in the position of nerves and foramina
- collateral nerve supply.

Bony barriers to diffusion

The diffusion of local anaesthetic solution to the pulpal supply to the teeth through bone is required for successful anaesthesia in techniques other than regional block, intraosseous and intraseptal methods. There are two ways diffusion may be affected. First, the presence of thick cortical bone can represent a barrier to the local anaesthetic. This is of course the reason why in

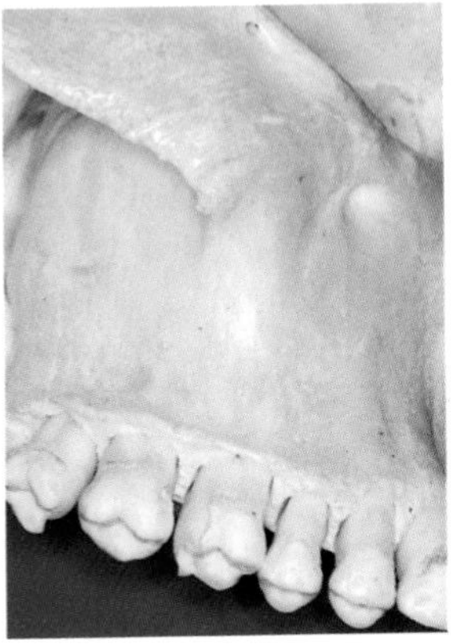

Fig 8-1 The zygomatic buttress can inhibit the infiltration of local anaesthetic solution after buccal deposition in the first molar region.

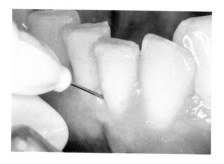

Fig 8-2 Intraligamentary anaesthesia is unreliable in the mandibular incisor region in adults.

the adult mandible regional block methods are used. This problem may also manifest itself in the maxilla where the thick zygomatic buttress can prevent diffusion of solution to the first maxillary molar tooth (Fig 8-1). This is overcome by injecting both mesial and distal to the buttress. The second method by which diffusion may be poor is during intraligamentary injections. This method relies upon entry of material via the perforations in the wall of the socket. In regions such as the mandibular anteriors there is a paucity of perforations in the socket and thus this technique is unreliable in this zone (Fig 8-2).

Variations in the position of nerves and foramina
The positions of foramina such as the mandibular and mental foramina are not consistent. In addition to variations with age there are also marked differences between patients. The mandibular foramen is often obvious on panoramic radiographs and if one of these is available it should be viewed before the administration of an inferior alveolar nerve block. The use of one of the methods, which does not rely on deposition close to the mandibular foramen such as the Akinosi or Gow-Gates techniques, can overcome the problem of an ectopic mandibular foramen. Unfortunately, the mental foramen is not always obvious on panoramic radiographs but may be shown in intraoral periapical films. Nevertheless, even when local anaesthetic solution is deposited at the site of the foramen using techniques such as ultra-sonic guidance, the success following inferior alveolar nerve blocks is not guaranteed. This supports the view that collateral nerve supply may be responsible for failure in some cases.

Collateral nerve supply
1. Maxilla
It is not only the superior alveolar nerves that supply the pulps of the maxillary teeth. In the maxilla the greater palatine and nasopalatine nerves may

contribute fibres to the pulps. Blocking these nerves or palatal infiltration injections close to the tooth in question may be required to obtain satisfactory maxillary pulpal anaesthesia.

2. Mandible

As is the case with the maxilla there is the potential for collateral supply in the mandibular pulps. Indeed, the problem may be more apparent in the mandible owing to the fact that the methods of anaesthesia used are regional blocks. Block anaesthesia is less likely to counter collateral supply compared with infiltration methods, which are normally used in the maxilla. The following accessory supply may be encountered:

- additional fibres from the ipsilateral inferior alveolar nerve
- fibres from the contralateral inferior alveolar nerve
- lingual nerve
- long buccal nerve
- mylohyoid nerve
- auriculotemporal nerve
- cervical nerves.

1. Additional fibres from the ipsilateral inferior alveolar nerve

It is possible that some fibres leave the inferior alveolar nerve proximal to the mandibular foramen and enter the bone through accessory foramina (Figs 8-3a,b and 8-4). If the point of separation from the main nerve is proximal

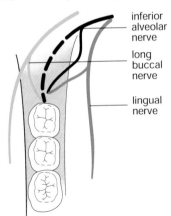

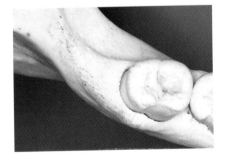

Fig 8-3a The area distal to the lower third molar may contain an anastomosis of nerves that can provide accessory pulpal supply.

Fig 8-3b Perforations in the mandibular retromolar area may allow passage of nerves providing accessory supply to the pulps of the mandibular teeth.

113

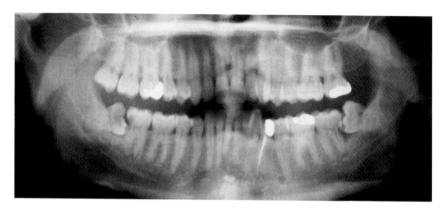

Fig 8-4 A radiograph showing a distinct canal in the retromolar region.

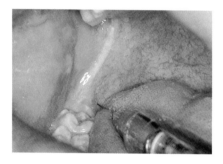

Fig 8-5 Depositing solution in the retromolar area may help nullify accessory nerve supply in this region.

to the mandibular foramen then a standard inferior alveolar nerve block may not reach the accessory supply. This problem will be countered by giving a "high" block such as the Gow-Gates or Akinosi methods. Another useful place to deposit solution is directly in the retromolar region just lingual to the third molar (Fig 8-5). This will counter any supply reaching this zone from the inferior alveolar, lingual and long buccal nerves.

2. Fibres from the contralateral inferior alveolar nerve
Midline structures can obtain bilateral nerve supply. Thus, the mandibular incisors may obtain supply from both inferior alveolar nerves. Such supply may be countered by infiltration anaesthesia (both buccal and lingual). Fortunately, infiltration anaesthesia is successful in the mandibular incisor region.

114

3. Lingual nerve
The lingual nerve may supply the pulps of the mandibular teeth. Normally, approaches to the inferior alveolar nerve will anaesthetise the lingual nerve. Additionally, lingual infiltration injections adjacent to the tooth of interest can be used.

4. The long buccal nerve
Supply from the long buccal nerve may contribute to the pulp. The point of entry of the accessory fibres into the bone governs the method of countering this supply. If the nerve enters the bone through the buccal alveolus then a buccal infiltration should suffice. If the point of entry is in the retromolar region (Fig 8-3) then a true long buccal block will be required.

5. The mylohyoid nerve
The mylohyoid nerve separates from the inferior alveolar nerve almost 15 mm from the mandibular foramen. It travels lingual to the mandible and may send accessory fibres to the pulps through the lingual mandibular cortex (Fig 8-6). Therefore, it may not be affected by a standard inferior alveolar nerve block. The use of lingual infiltration adjacent to the tooth of interest, a

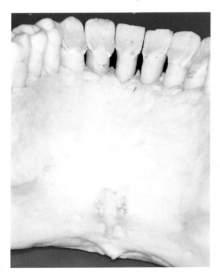

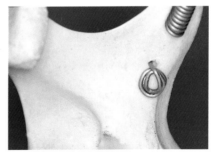

Fig 8-6 The lingual cortex of the mandible has many perforations that may allow accessory nerve supply to the pulps from sources such as the mylohyoid nerve.

Fig 8-7 Perforations high in the ramus may permit fibres from the auriculotemporal nerve to reach the pulps of the teeth.

115

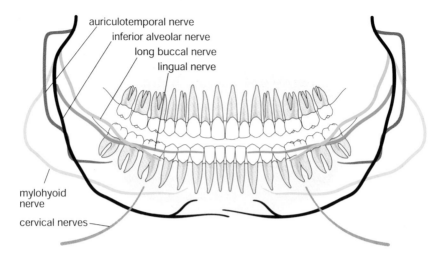

auriculotemporal nerve
inferior alveolar nerve
long buccal nerve
lingual nerve

mylohyoid
nerve

cervical nerves

Fig 8-8 A summary of the potential accessory nerves supplying the teeth.

mylohyoid nerve block, or the Akinosi or Gow-Gates methods can be used to counter mylohyoid nerve supply.

<u>6. The auriculotemporal nerve</u>
The auriculotemporal nerve may supply the pulps of the teeth via fibres that enter the mandible in the condylar region or adjacent parts of the superior ramus (Fig 8-7). The only techniques that could nullify this supply are the "high" blocks - namely, the Akinosi and Gow-Gates methods.

<u>7. Cervical nerves</u>
The Gow-Gates method should counter all accessory supply from the ipsilateral mandibular nerve. Unfortunately, this method is not 100% successful even in experienced hands. One explanation for failure is that fibres from nerves other than the mandibular nerve are contributing to pulpal supply. It is possible that the upper cervical nerves can provide pulpal supply to the teeth. This can be overcome by buccal and lingual infiltration adjacent to the tooth of interest.

The accessory supplies to the mandibular teeth are summarised in Fig 8-8.

Use of supplementary techniques to overcome failure due to collateral supply
Intraosseous, intraligamentary and intrapulpal anaesthesia may be used to counter accessory nerve supply, as these techniques are independent of the

origin of the nerve. Certainly, the combination of intraosseous or intraligamentary anaesthesia with inferior alveolar nerve blocks increases efficacy compared with the regional block method alone. Unfortunately, as mentioned above, the intraligamentary route is not successful in all sites; it is poor in obtaining pulpal anaesthesia of lower incisors.

Pathological Causes of Failure

Two pathological conditions can cause problems with anaesthesia - namely, trismus and inflammation.

Trismus

Trismus leading to inability to reach the area of needle penetration may contribute to failure. The methods used to overcome this problem were discussed above.

Inflammation

A number of explanations have been suggested as to why inflamed teeth are resistant to anaesthesia. One practical problem is that the presence of a draining sinus can lead to escape of injected solution intraorally, which means it does not diffuse to the site of action. It has been suggested that inflammation decreases the pH in the tissues and therefore the lipophillic moiety of the local anaesthetic agent is present in reduced concentration, so there is less to enter the nerve and produce conduction blockade. In addition, it has been suggested that the presence of hyperaemia increases the washout of the local anaesthetic, thus reducing efficacy (Fig 8-9). The pH and hyperaemia hypotheses might help to explain why infiltrations are ineffective in the presence of inflammation. These theories do not explain the failure of block tech-

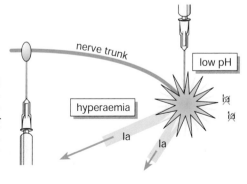

Fig 8-9 It has been suggested that hyperaemia and low pH in the presence of inflammation are reasons for failure in the presence of pulpitis. If that were the case then regional block anaesthesia would always be successful in such a circumstance. Unfortunately, this is not so.

niques where the solution has been deposited distant to the inflamed tissues. The explanation is that inflamed nerves are hyperalgesic - in other words, they transmit impulses under minimal stimulation. The way to overcome this is to inject more local anaesthetic. It is analogous to treating mild hunger with a snack but starvation with a large meal. If sufficient solution is deposited in the correct place then anaesthesia will eventually occur. The proof is that too much local anaesthesia will eventually produce general anaesthesia. It is therefore important when dealing with failure owing to inflammation that due consideration is given to the maximum doses suggested in Chapter 7. It has been demonstrated that the use of more concentrated anaesthetic solutions, such as 5% lidocaine, can overcome failure in cases of hyperalgesia. This solution is not available in dental local anaesthetic cartridges. The alternative is to inject more of the standard solution while remaining within the safe maximum dose schedule. This may involve using technique combinations such as intraligamentary, infiltration and regional block methods.

Pharmaceutical Causes of Failure

The solutions supplied by local anaesthetic manufacturers are of a high quality and when properly stored there should be no pharmaceutical cause of failure. Improper storage may decrease efficacy. For example, keeping cartridges at high temperature or in light may lead to loss of activity of epinephrine, which will decrease effectiveness.

Pharmacological Causes of Failure

There are some possible interactions between drugs and local anaesthetics. These may cause failure owing to more rapid elimination or metabolism of the anaesthetic. These are theoretical rather than of clinical importance. In this regard it is worth mentioning that reversal of local anaesthesia is possible by injection of alpha-adrenergic agonists but at present this is not recommended. These agents achieve their effect by reversing epinephrine-induced vasoconstriction.

The most likely cause of pharmacological failure is the injection of too small a dose. This may explain why a repeat injection often overcomes failure.

Psychological Causes of Failure

Anaesthesia is more successful in relaxed patients. This means that conscious sedation may be useful in overcoming failure in some cases. Conscious sedation is not an alternative to good local anaesthesia; it should be used in conjunction with excellent pain control. Conscious sedation offers a number of advantages in relation to the administration of local anaesthesia. These include:

• anxiolysis
• reducing needle phobia
• producing muscle relaxation
• overcoming gagging
• providing pharmacological protection
• producing analgesia.

As well as relaxing the patient, which increases success, conscious sedation may make the receipt of multiple injections more acceptable. As mentioned above, multiple injections are often the key to overcoming failure. Conscious sedation may also allow the use of local anaesthesia in needle-phobic patients, some of who will accept injections in the hand but have concerns over intraoral needle penetration. Conscious sedation may overcome trismus due to muscle tension and prevent gagging which can lead to failure due to inability to locate the needle properly. In addition, with some drug combinations there is protection against toxicity. For example, midazolam decreases the CNS toxicity of lidocaine. Finally, relative analgesia can reduce the discomfort of injections. This may be particularly useful in children.

Technical Causes of Failure

The success of local anaesthesia is technique dependent. Failure owing to poor technique may be improved by practice or by the choice of an appropriate alternative method.

The Approach to the Failed Case

Methods of dealing with failure of anaesthesia in both jaws are illustrated diagrammatically in Figs 8-10 and 8-11. Multiple injections cannot be avoided and it is important to reinforce the point that the maximum recommended doses must not be exceeded. The decision as to how much solution can be injected safely in a particular patient must be made before the first injection is given. This decision should not be overruled. The time to perform mental arithmetic is not halfway through a session when the situation is getting out of control. If the predetermined amount of local anaesthetic is not successful then it is safer to halt proceedings and try again another day or refer to a colleague.

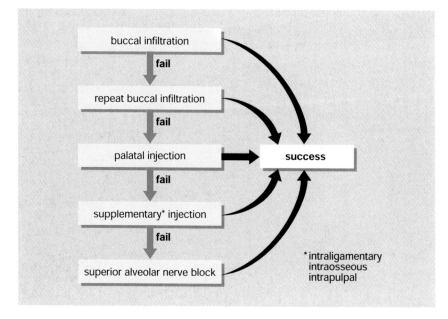

Fig 8-10 A flow diagram outlining the approach to failed injections in the upper jaw.

Post-anaesthetic Problems

A number of problems may occur following dental local anaesthesia. Some of these, such as hemifacial paralysis, are discussed in Chapter 7. Other post-injection problems include:
• bleeding
• pain
• prolonged altered sensation
• trismus
• infection.

Bleeding

Bleeding may occur at the site of mucosal penetration when the needle is removed. This is rarely dramatic and manual pressure for a few minutes is normally effective. Bleeding in deeper tissues may be more problematic and it is for this reason that deep block injections must be avoided in patients with bleeding diathesis such as haemophilia, unless appropriate prophylaxis has been provided.

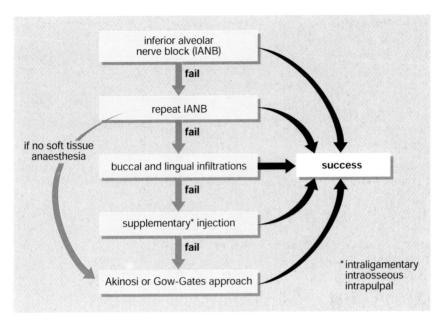

Fig 8-11 A flow diagram outlining the approach to failed injections in the lower jaw.

Pain

Periosteal stripping and tissue damage may cause pain after injection. In addition, inappropriate forces during intraligamentary anaesthesia can extrude a tooth from its socket leading to occlusal trauma. Methods used to reduce pain during injection are described in the Chapter 9. Many of these techniques will help to reduce post-operative discomfort - for example, ensuring that the needle is not sub-periosteal will prevent raising of the periosteum from the bone. Slow injection will limit soft tissue trauma and prevent tooth extrusion during intraligamentary anaesthesia.

Self-inflicted trauma can produce painful lesions in the area of anaesthesia. The patient, and in the case of a child the parent, should be advised about the avoidance of trauma to the area during the period of anaesthesia.

Pain may also be produced as a result of injury to the nerve. Damage to the nerve by the needle may also produce prolonged altered sensation.

Prolonged altered sensation

Prolonged anaesthesia or paraesthesia may be the result of physical or chemical damage to a nerve trunk. Unfortunately, trauma from the needle to the nerve is not always preventable. When the patient's reaction suggests direct contact with the nerve during an injection then solution should not be injected at that point. This will produce further damage. In this event the needle should be withdrawn slightly before solution is deposited.

Nerve damage following regional block injections appears to be more likely when local anaesthetic concentration is increased. Thus, the more concentrated solutions are best avoided when regional blocks are being used.

There is very little that can be done for the patient with prolonged altered sensation following local anaesthesia. Reassurance that the condition should resolve should be provided. In addition, the patient must be reviewed until normal sensation returns to ensure that no damage is occurring in the anaesthetised region.

Trismus

Trismus may occur following regional block methods to anaesthetise the inferior alveolar, posterior superior alveolar or maxillary nerves. Occasionally, posterior maxillary infiltrations may also produce trismus. The condition is the result of muscle spasm that may be owing to bleeding following the penetration of a deep vessel. Alternatively, direct injection of local anaesthetic solution into a muscle might produce spasm. Ensuring that bony contact has been achieved and depositing solution just supraperiosteally may avoid injection into muscle.

When trismus occurs, the patient should be reassured that jaw function will return to normal but that it may take a few weeks. If a large haematoma is obvious and is at risk of infection, a short dose of antibiotics may be useful. Such a prescription is not advised in the absence of a large haematoma.

Infection

The transfer of infected material to the patient should never occur when proper cross-infection measures are implemented. The use of sterilised equipment and the avoidance of needlestick injury are essential. Materials should not be used beyond their expiry date and should be stored under appropriate conditions to avoid microbial contamination. It is thought that local anaesthetic injections may activate latent viral infections such as *Herpes*. This is because ulceration is noted occasionally at the site of injection. This would appear to be a rare occurrence.

Conclusions

- Local anaesthesia may produce problems before and after injection.
- Most unwanted effects are not serious.
- Failure of anaesthesia is an occupational hazard.
- Understanding the reasons for failure helps overcome this problem.

Further Reading

Haas DA, Lennon D. A 21-year retrospective study of reports of paresthesia following local anesthetic administration. J Canad Dent Assoc 1995;61:319-330

Hannan L, Reader A, Nist R, Beck M, Meyers WJ. The use of ultrasound for guiding needle placement for inferior alveolar nerve blocks. Oral Surg Oral Med Oral Path 1999;87:658-665.

Heasman PA, Beynon ADG. Clinical anatomy of regional analgesia: An approach to failure. Dent Update 1986;Nov/Dec:469-476.

Chapter 9
Painless Local Anaesthesia: Is It Possible?

Aim

The aim of this chapter is to consider factors that influence the discomfort of dental local anaesthetic injections.

Outcome

After reading this chapter you should have an understanding of the factors that produce pain during local anaesthesia in dentistry and appreciate techniques that can reduce injection sensation.

Introduction

It is unfortunate that the methods used to control dental operative pain may themselves produce discomfort. It should be the aim of all caring practitioners to reduce injection sensation to a minimum. The following factors can influence injection discomfort:
• the expectation of pain
• the needle
• the syringe
• the area of the mouth injected
• the technique
• the anaesthetic solution
• the order of injection.

The dentist can influence all of these factors and thus can control the degree of discomfort produced during intraoral injections. Each of these elements will be considered.

The expectation of pain

Patients with low pain expectancy experience less injection discomfort than those with a high pain expectancy. The belief that patients are going to receive a topical anaesthetic can reduce their pain expectancy. This means that suggestion can be used to reduce the pain experience. Taking this a stage further may involve formal hypnosis. Some patients can experience total pain control by hypnosis, in others the technique can be used to reduce injection discomfort.

The needle

As far as the patient is concerned, it is probably the needle that is the most obvious cause of pain. The use of systems such as jet injectors could eliminate the needle altogether. These devices are not 100% effective in reducing operative pain. Indeed, in some studies subjects report more discomfort with the use of jet injection compared to infiltration anaesthesia. Factors that could influence the pain produced by needle insertion include:

needle gauge
needle condition
surface preparation
relative analgesia.

Needle gauge

It might appear obvious that the narrower the gauge of the needle the less discomfort produced by the injection. There is no evidence in the dental literature that supports this view. The gauges used in dentistry in the UK (27 and 30) appear to produce the same amount of discomfort and thus needle selection within these gauges does not influence injection pain.

Needle condition

Dental needles are provided with sharp points to enable easy penetration of the tissues. When they have been used the point loses its sharpness

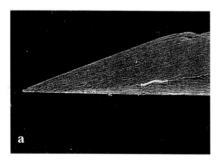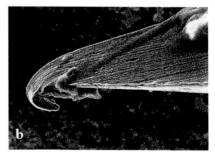

Fig 9-1 Scanning electron micrographs of an unused needle (9.1a) and a needle after contact with bone (9.1b). Note the deformation of the point after use. (Photographs kindly supplied by Dr John Rout).

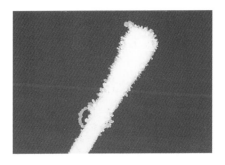

Fig 9-2 An iceball produced by spraying a cotton bud with ethyl chloride.

(Fig 9-1). Thus it would appear prudent to use a fresh needle for every tissue puncture.

Surface preparation
A number of methods of surface preparation may be employed. These include:
- refrigeration
- topical anaesthesia
- jet injection
- transcutaneous electronic nerve stimulation.

Refrigeration
The use of refrigeration has been suggested to reduce the discomfort of needle penetration in the palate. The tissue is treated for 5 seconds with an ice ball prior to needle insertion. Treating a cotton pellet with a volatile liquid, such as ethyl chloride, produces the ice ball (Fig 9-2).

Topical anaesthesia
Topical anaesthetics may have both a psychological and a pharmacological effect. It was mentioned above that the suggestion that a topical anaesthetic will be used reduces pain expectation. Is this the only benefit or do topicals produce a pharmacological benefit? There is evidence that topical anaesthetics do produce a pharmacological effect. As discussed in Chapter 6, the following factors influence the pharmacological efficacy of topical anaesthetics:
- the agent selected
- the duration of application
- the site of application.

The topical anaesthetic agent
There is evidence that anaesthetic agents are better than placebo at reducing injection discomfort. In addition, not all anaesthetic agents show the same efficacy. A dose response has been demonstrated with lidocaine. For example, patches containing 20% lidocaine are more effective than those containing 10% lidocaine. In addition, the eutectic mixture of lidocaine and prilocaine has been shown to be more effective than lidocaine alone. Unfortunately, this preparation is not licensed for intraoral use at present.

The duration of application
In order to achieve a pharmacological effect, the topical anaesthetic must be present for more than a brief application An application time of five minutes may be required to ensure a pharmacological effect.

The site of application
Topical anaesthetics will achieve an effect in the maxillary and mandibular buccal mucosa after a five-minute application. Efficacy on highly keratinised tissue such as palatal mucosa is not as good. In addition, there is no evidence that topical anaesthetics achieve any benefit in reducing the discomfort of deep regional block injections such as inferior alveolar nerve blocks (Fig 9-3).

Jet injection
Jet injectors may be used as the definitive method of anaesthesia or they can be employed to allow pain-free needle penetration. They have been shown to reduce the discomfort of subsequent needle penetration, although this effect is not universal.

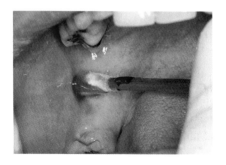

Fig 9-3 There is no evidence that topical anaesthetics produce any relief of discomfort prior to deep regional block injections.

Transcutaneous electronic nerve stimulation
Transcutaneous electronic nerve stimulation (TENS), which is a form of electroanalgesia, can be used both as a means of anaesthetising teeth and a method of reducing injection pain. This technique has been shown to reduce injection discomfort. In addition to reducing the discomfort of infiltration anaesthesia, TENS has been demonstrated to reduce the pain of deep regional block injections such as inferior alveolar nerve blocks (Fig 6-13). The technique can be cumbersome and some patients may be anxious about the concept of having electrodes in their mouth!

Relative analgesia
As the name suggests, relative analgesia has pain-reducing properties. This method can reduce the discomfort of dental local anaesthesia including the pain of deep regional block injections.

The syringe
As mentioned above, the expectation of pain influences the discomfort experienced. Different designs of syringe produce different levels of anxiety in patients. The pistol grip type of intraligamentary syringe has been shown to produce more anxiety than computerised delivery systems.

In addition, as intravascular injections can produce palpitations and other systemic effects that may be unpleasant, every effort should be made to avoid such events by using a syringe that permits aspiration.

The area of the mouth injected
It is obvious to anyone who administers dental local anaesthetics that different areas of the mouth vary in the pain experienced during injection. Regional block injections produce more discomfort than infiltration techniques and intraligamentary injections can be more uncomfortable than infiltrations. Palatal injections are more unpleasant than buccal infiltrations.

The technique
The main factor relating to technique that influences injection discomfort is the speed of delivery. The faster the injection, the more uncomfortable it is for the patient. The use of very slow delivery speeds, perhaps by the use of computerised delivery systems, reduces injection discomfort. It cannot be overemphasised that slow administration is the cornerstone to success no matter which technique or type of equipment is chosen. There is no avoiding the fact that pain-free anaesthesia is time-consuming.

The anaesthetic solution

Solution-dependent factors that influence injection discomfort include:
• temperature
• pH.

Temperature

Patients are unable to differentiate differences in temperature between 15°C and body temperature. Therefore, as long as the cartridge has been stored at room temperature, there is no need to heat it prior to use. When cartridges are stored in a refrigerator then they should be allowed to reach room temperature before injection. It is unwise to store cartridges at body temperature for a prolonged time before use. Storage at higher temperatures produces a number of unwanted effects including:
• increasing the chances of bacterial contamination
• reducing the efficacy of epinephrine
• decreasing the pH of the solution.

pH

Local anaesthetic solutions have different pHs. Epinephrine-containing anaesthetics have lower pHs than plain solutions. These differences in pH produce different injection sensations: the lower the pH the more uncomfortable the injection. Epinephrine-containing solutions are preferred for pulpal anaesthesia. If minimal discomfort is intended then an initial injection with an epinephrine-free anaesthetic can be followed with the definitive epinephrine-containing solution into the already anaesthetised zone.

The order of the injection

The order in which injections are given at the same visit affects perceived discomfort. If two identical injections are given to a patient on opposite sides of the mouth, the second injection is usually reported to be the more uncomfortable.

Technique for Painless Anaesthesia

When the factors considered above are taken into account, it is apparent that the best chance of administering a painless injection is at the first needle penetration. A site at which a painless injection may be given is therefore the ideal area to deliver the first dose. In the maxilla this is usually possible in the buccal sulcus, particularly in the premolar and molar region. Once a zone of anaesthesia has been obtained after the first injection, subsequent injections can be administered in the already anaesthetised area in a pain-free fashion.

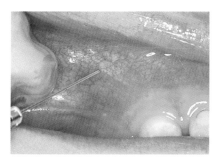

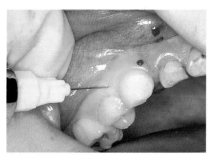

Fig 9-4a A buccal infiltration prior to an intrapapillary injection.

Fig 9-4b An intrapapillary injection chasing the anaesthetic through towards the palatal mucosa.

Fig 9-4c Palatal tissues blanch as the local anaesthetic is chased through from the buccal papilla.

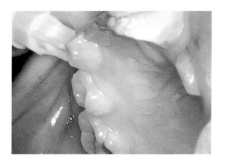

This is the so-called "chasing" technique. The following method is suggested in the maxilla. If the tooth of interest is an anterior tooth, the initial injection is best given in the premolar region (Fig 9-4a). After waiting one minute, further buccal injections are given more anteriorly and chased around to the tooth of interest (Fig 9-4). The steps are as follows:

1. Apply topical anaesthesia in the appropriate zone of the buccal sulcus for 5 minutes.
2. After removing the topical anaesthetic, stretch the mucosa in the area to be injected so that it is taut.
3. Pierce the tense mucosa with a new needle and advance to a subepithelial but supraperiosteal position (Fig 9-4a).
4. Aspirate.

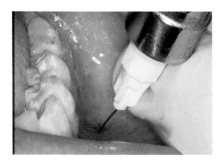

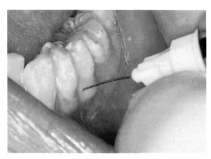

Fig 9-5a A buccal infiltration prior to a buccal intrapapillary injection.

Fig 9-5b The buccal intrapapillary injection prior to an intraligamentary injection.

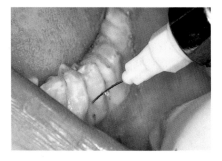

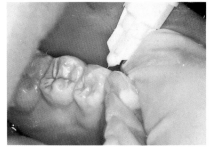

Fig 9-5c The intraligamentary injection.

Fig 9-5d Blanching of the lingual tissues during the intraligamentary injection on the buccal side. This often occurs in children. This may indicate satisfactory lingual anaesthesia although a separate lingual intraligamentary injection may be given.

5. Inject slowly, either manually at a rate of 1 mL/30seconds or using a computerised delivery system.
6. If palatal anaesthesia is required, this is obtained by injecting into the buccal papilla and administering a papillary injection once the buccal infiltration has achieved anaesthesia (Fig 9-4b). A short 12 mm needle is ideal for this technique. The needle is advanced slowly, while still injecting, through the papilla to the palatal side and by this method solution is de-

posited in the palatal mucosa (Fig 9-4c). Blanching of the palatal tissues indicates successful deposition in the palate. It is advisable to have an aspirator in place at the palatal side in the zone being entered. This is because if the palatal mucosa is breached during needle advancement the aspirator will collect any solution that may be injected into the mouth. Local anaesthetics are wonderful drugs, but they taste awful. This may be all that is needed to produce palatal anaesthesia, although a needle can be inserted within the blanched zone and anaesthesia chased to other areas of the palate. When injecting into the palate in this way a computerised delivery system is useful in reducing injection sensation.

In the mandible it is difficult to anaesthetise the full depth of tissue penetration prior to regional block injections. Using an electronic delivery system and injecting as the needle advances through tissue to the point of interest can be performed with minimal discomfort. In the deciduous dentition, and in adult anterior teeth, the method of choice in the mandible is infiltration anaesthesia and the technique described for the maxilla can be employed. If extracting mandibular premolar teeth in children, the best method of obtaining pain-free anaesthesia is to follow a buccal infiltration with a papillary injection, which then allows pain-free intraligamentary anaesthesia that can be chased through to the lingual side (Figs 9-5a-d).

To Answer the Question

The title of this chapter posed the question "painless anaesthesia - is it possible?" The answer is "yes" - for many of the techniques used in dentistry. Certainly it should be possible in the maxilla. The methods used to achieve pain-free anaesthesia are time-consuming and present a challenge to both dentist and patient. Both parties must work as a team. When the goal is achieved, the dentist obtains satisfaction and the patient has improved quality of care. The extra time spent is well worth the effort.

Conclusions

- Dentists can influence a number of factors governing injection discomfort.
- Careful choice of equipment and technique can reduce injection discomfort.
- Painless anaesthesia *is* possible.

Further Reading

Hersh EV, Houpt MI, Cooper SA, Feldman RS, Wolff MS, Levin LM. Analgesic efficacy and safety of an intraoral lidocaine patch. J Amer Dent Assoc 1996;127:1626-634.

Meechan JG. Intraoral topical anaesthetics. A review. J Dent 2000;28:3-14.

Wilson S, Molina L de L, Preisch J, Weaver J. The effect of electronic dental anesthesia on behavior during local anesthetic injection in the young, sedated dental patient. Paed Dent 1999;21:12-17.

Index

A

B

Quintessentials for General Dental Practitioners Series

in 36 volumes

Editor-in-Chief: Professor Nairn H F Wilson

The Quintessentials for General Dental Practitioners Series covers basic principles and key issues in all aspects of modern dental medicine. Each book can be read as a stand-alone volume or in conjunction with other books in the series.

Publication date, approximately

Oral Surgery and Oral Medicine, Editor: John G Meechan

Practical Dental Local Anaesthesia	available
Practical Oral Medicine	Spring 2004
Practical Conscious Sedation	Autumn 2003
Practical Surgical Dentistry	Spring 2004

Imaging, Editor: Keith Horner

Interpreting Dental Radiographs	available
Panoramic Radiology	Autumn 2003
Twenty-first Century Dental Imaging	Autumn 2004

Periodontology, Editor: Iain L C Chapple

Understanding Periodontal Diseases: Assessment and Diagnostic Procedures in Practice	available
Decision-Making for the Periodontal Team	Autumn 2003
Successful Periodontal Therapy – A Non-Surgical Approach	Autumn 2003
Periodontal Management of Children and Adolescents	Autumn 2003
Periodontal Medicine in Practice	Spring 2004

Implantology, Editor: Lloyd J Searson

Implants for the General Practitioner	available
Managing Orofacial Pain in General Dental Practice	Spring 2003

Endodontics, Editor: John M Whitworth

Rational Root Canal Treatment in Practice	available
Managing Endodontic Failure in Practice	Autumn 2003
Managing Dental Trauma in Practice	Autumn 2003
Managing the Vital Pulp in Practice	Autumn 2004

Prosthodontics, Editor: P Finbarr Allen

Teeth for Life for Older Adults	available
Complete Dentures – from Planning to Problem Solving	Autumn 2003
Removable Partial Dentures – A Systematic Approach	Autumn 2003
Fixed Prosthodontics for the General Dental Practitioner	Autumn 2003
Occlusion: A Theoretical and Team Approach	Autumn 2004

Operative Dentistry, Editor: Paul A Brunton

Decision-Making in Operative Dentistry	available
Applied Dental Materials in Operative Dentistry	Spring 2003
Aesthetic Dentistry	Autumn 2003
Successful Indirect Restorations in General Practice	Spring 2004

Paediatric Dentistry/Orthodontics, Editor: Marie Therese Hosey

Child Taming: How to Cope with Children in Dental Practice	Spring 2003
Paediatric Cariology	Autumn 2003
Treatment Planning for the Developing Dentition	Autumn 2003

General Dentistry and Practice Management, Editor: Raj Rattan

The Business of Dentistry	available
Risk Management in General Dental Practice	Spring 2003
Practice Management for the Dental Team	Autumn 2003
Application of Information Technology in General Dental Practice	Spring 2004
Quality Assurance in General Dental Practice	Autumn 2004
Evidence-Based Care in General Dental Practice	Spring 2005

Quintessence Publishing Co. Ltd., London